MW01534326

Stroke Victims Have Rights
All About Strokes and Recovery

Also by Marlys J. Waters

NON-FICTION

There Must Be an Easier Way to Die
Surrounded by Tragedy, The Life of Harold Launspach
Wetter-Miller-Schneider-Riedesel Families, Genealogy
Hickory's Journey, Lost Pig Finds a New Home
Nemaha, Iowa Centennial Book 1999, 2nd Edition
His Spirit Fights Back, The Premature Death Of Steven Lee
    Hatch 7/13/1948 – 8/6/2015
Shortcut to Heaven, Why Death-With-Dignity Legislation is
    Needed Now
Stroke Victims Have Rights, All About Strokes and Recovery

FICTION

The Congressman's Demise, A Marsha Walters Mystery

MUSIC BOOKS

Music Flashback Vol 1: Ragtime, Jazz & Boogie Woogie
Music Flashback Vol 2: Ragtime, Jazz & Boogie Woogie

Stroke Victims Have Rights
All About Strokes and Recovery

By Marlys J. Waters

Power of the Pen Publishing
Nemaha, Iowa

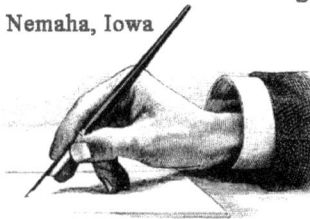

© 2016 by Marlys J. Waters

All rights reserved. No part of this book may be shared, reproduced or utilized in any form or by any means, electronic or mechanical, including photocopying, recording or by any information storage and retrieval system, without permission in writing from the Publisher. Inquiries should be addressed to Permissions Department, Power of the Pen Publishing, PO Box 5, Nemaha, IA 50567

First Edition

ISBN-13: 978-1530787586
ISBN-10: 1530787580

Printed in the United States of America

Table of Contents

Introduction

This book was written to show how ignorant the majority of medical professionals, family, and caregivers are regarding a person who has suffered a stroke and is unable to speak. The victim becomes isolated from a talking world whose members have no idea how to communicate with a person that can not make his voice respond to his commands. They don't even realize there is an active, normal mind inside that head crying to be heard but without the ability to verbalize his thoughts.

The man whose ordeal and subsequent death that sparked the writing of this book was my 12-year companion -- Steven Lee Hatch. He was 66 years old when he suffered a stroke on June 21, 2015 leaving him paralyzed on his right side, and unable to speak or to swallow. He died a month and a half later of medical incompetence and neglect.

Side affects of one-sided paralysis, loss of speech, and inability to swallow are typical for most stroke victims that live through the initial blood clot or ruptured artery that damaged part of their brain. Most people not only survive but regain part or full use of their paralyzed limbs, their ability to swallow, and a return back to their prior life with possibly a small but lingering speech impediment or other small disability.

Steve Hatch did not get the care and rehabilitation he needed and was forced into Hospice and taken out of skilled nursing care without his permission a month after his stroke. He died age 67 on August 6, 2015 – less than seven weeks after the stroke and only 13 days after being illegally placed into Hospice.

Included are stories of movie stars and other public persons who have released their disability to the public to assist in a better understanding of their life and healing after their stroke and their successful return to public life. The thinking part of the mind usually remains intact, the soul of your loved one is the same. All they need to recover is the ability to let you know they are still the same person, their personality and sense of humor remain, they are just temporarily quiet.

I was the only person who knew Steve's mind was fine and that he wanted me to take him home and give him the care and rehabilitation he needed. Steve had ample Medicare and Supplemental Insurance to pay 100% for his care, treatment, therapy, and rehabilitation for up to 90 days and partial care after that time. He had other resources, he was not destitute and could have hired the best stroke rehabilitation professionals. But the medical profession just chalked him off as a vegetable.

Steve Hatch was stuck in a nursing home which didn't offer the specialized stroke rehab he needed. I was not allowed access to any of his medical records or updates on his care or progress since I wasn't family. He was not able to tell me anything during my 2-4 hour daily visits at the hospitals and in the care center. I did not know he wasn't receiving the care he needed until they placed him into hospice.

Hospice told his estranged brother that he was dying and had the brother sign the papers authorizing hospice. Medicare required him to be taken out of skilled nursing care and stroke rehabilitation in order to be covered under hospice. Yet Steve's condition had not changed on July 24, 2015 when hospice took over. He had a good chance for partial to full recovery with me as his full-time experienced caregiver along with home health care nurses.

Steve died only 13 days after being administered palliative medications for pain (he had no pain), depression (there was no depression), and sleep (he had no trouble sleeping). His body was unable to survive without the curative medications he had been taking for long-term ailments but which were replaced with sedatives/morphine that hospice injected into him as he lay in bed at the care center. He went into a coma on the 12th day of hospice and died the next morning.

The purpose of this book is to disclose the rights of the stroke victim, a timeline for the expected recovery process, and a technical description of the physical changes that occur in your head and body.

There is life after stroke, it might be different than before but it can be fun if the victim has someone to assist with their rehabilitation. Steve Hatch and I would have had a future designing equipment for him to test, making up exercises to improve his speech, swallowing, and movement of his paralyzed side, and researching the best equipment to help him get around. Steve had an insight and mechanical understanding of what makes things tick. He would have been the perfect person to test prototypes and inventions. While he was unable to speak, he had an uncanny knowledge of computer use and would have easily adapted to electronic communicating equipment using a touch screen. But he wasn't given the opportunity.

This book offers the stroke victim a Bill of Rights that you are entitled to use to fight for partial or full recovery. If you want to give up, hospice would be more than happy to assist you in a comfortable "death by sleeping". The choice is yours.

I've included stories of stroke survivors who were given the long-term care they needed and lived to tell about their experiences. They did not want to die and neither did Steven Lee Hatch.

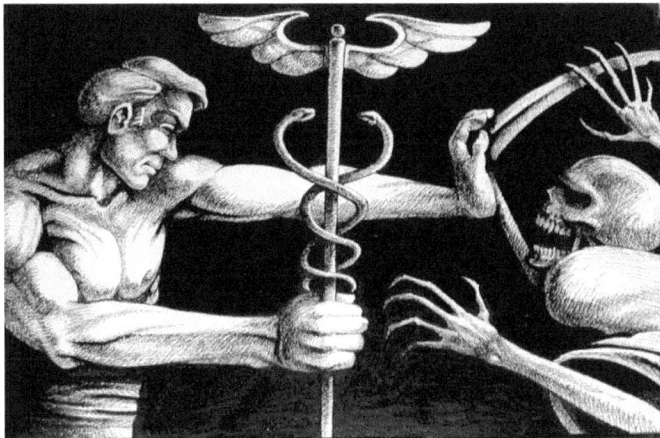

Stroke Victims Bill of Rights

1) **You have a right to make your own decisions.** As long as you are conscious and are able to answer "yes" or "no" to simple questions (or nod your head), you are in charge. The caregivers who have never seen you before are not allowed to assume your mind is not functioning just because you can't speak. Have your family member or friend state in writing that you need to be asked before decisions are made on any changes in your care or therapy. It is best if the caregivers (nurses, doctors, aides, hospice representatives) allow you to have a witness during their questioning on changes to your status/care and to record your answers.

2) **You have a right for intense stroke therapy and rehabilitation as soon as possible after the bleeding/clot has been stabilized**. Intense therapy and rehabilitation has the best chance for success when started within a week after your stroke. Laying on your back inert without physical and mental stimulation will not only slow down your recovery but might interfere with portions of the healing that can't be recovered later.

3) **You have a right for a family member or friend to work with you during your therapy.** They will be the ones taking care of you when you return home. They need to be taught (unless they are already experienced caregivers) on how to help you exercise, learn to make words, and exercises for swallowing. They can request the director of the hospital/care center to question you verbally on whether this person has your permission to be involved in your care and decision making (questions to you requiring yes or no answers only.). Don't let them say it must be in writing, a witness can put your response in writing but you have the authority to make the decision yourself even if you can't sign your name.

4) **You have a right to request being moved to a different nursing home/care center for specialized stroke**

rehabilitation. If your first placement after you leave the hospital is not giving you the care you need, you can be moved immediately, no waiting period required. They had their chance to show what they could offer you. If their care is grossly lacking, get out – move on.

5) **You may request a specialized wheel chair for your own use. It will be available for you only.** There are slightly reclining wheel chairs with head rests and side supports designed for paralyzed people with weakened neck muscles. You will quickly tire if you are wheeled to the therapy room or to the public areas or even set outside on a nice day without head support. It will be hard to not only hold your head upright but you will tend to slide/lean toward your paralyzed side no matter how many soft pillows they stuff against the armrest.

6) **You have a right to request any specialized equipment that will help in your rehabilitation and therapy.** Some extras will probably be at your expense or your insurance company may authorize their use. If your eyes are working fairly well, you might be able to communicate with the caregivers using your good hand via an electronic touch-screen notepad. They make them for people who are unable to verbalize their needs and come with pictures to touch which will speak for you.

7) **You have a right to request exercise equipment that you can use yourself.** One of the simplest gadgets that stroke wards at hospitals use is a large ring suspended over the bed that you can reach with your active hand. That gives you the opportunity to lift and slightly move your shoulder if you want to adjust your position. There are other simple exercise devices which can be used for not only your good side but passive gizmos that might be used to improve the blood flow to your paralyzed side which will stimulate nerve regeneration. See the chapter on "Inventions and Aids for Stroke Victims".

8) **Everyone needs emotional stimulation.** If you don't have a family member or friend nearby, there needs to be a caring volunteer assigned who would be willing to make daily visits to read to you, to chat about the weather, to inquire about your care. This person can become your advocate and will learn to read your responses even if the words don't make sense. They can speak to your legal advisor if they detect something isn't right in your care. They can also tell you about life after you are released from the care/rehabilitation center. How about an electric wheel chair which you can use on the sidewalk by your home? How about a gym in your garage filled with equipment you only dreamed of? Want to play a musical instrument? Some can be operated with only one hand, others can be blown into which might improve your throat muscles. See something lacking in your assigned touch screen program? Time for you to start inventing better programs and equipment. Your mind is still active, so use it!

9) **If you left a pet at home, your family should be encouraged to bring the dog or cat to visit you.** If that isn't allowed, maybe it is time to move back home or to a different care center. You lost everything after your stroke when you were taken out of your home, away from your work and hobbies. You will heal faster physically if your emotional needs are also met.

10) **You have a right to expect caregivers and visitors to accept you as you are.** People who have never seen a stroke victim need to be given advanced instruction so they don't hurt your feelings when they see you drooling out the paralyzed side of your mouth, or to not answer their questions because it requires multiple words that you are unable to verbalize. Some will think you have no mind. Your advocate needs to educate people on the dark side of strokes or to read this book. Your friends who understand what you are going through emotionally will be able to accept you as you are and cheer you up. Those who find

your droopy face disgusting or your motionless body repulsive weren't your friends and you don't need them. And shame on the doctor who calls you a "vegetable" as he needs to go into a different profession immediately. This book will give you descriptions and photos on what to expect of the paralyzed person. Don't give up on the stroke victim, the person you knew and loved is still inside that shell, the body has changed but the mind with personality and humor is till the same.

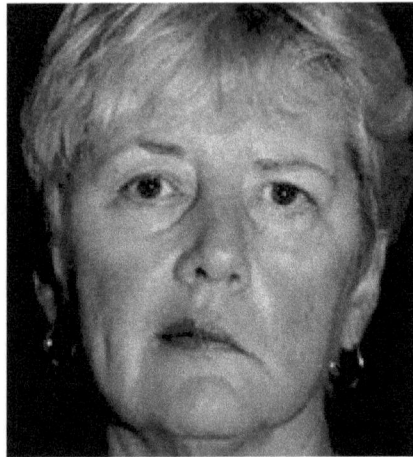

↬Lady with partially paralyzed face.

Signs of Stroke

The American Stroke Association advises everyone to learn to recognize these signs of stroke:

- Sudden numbness or weakness of the face, arm or leg, especially on one side of the body
- Sudden confusion, trouble speaking or understanding
- Sudden trouble seeing in one or both eyes
- Sudden trouble walking, dizziness, loss of balance or coordination
- Sudden, severe headache with no known cause

F.A.S.T.

The acronym FAST is an easy way to remember signs of stroke and what to do if you think a stroke has occurred. (The most important is to immediately call 9-1-1 for emergency assistance.) FAST stands for:

- **FACE.** Ask the person to smile. Check to see if one side of the face droops.

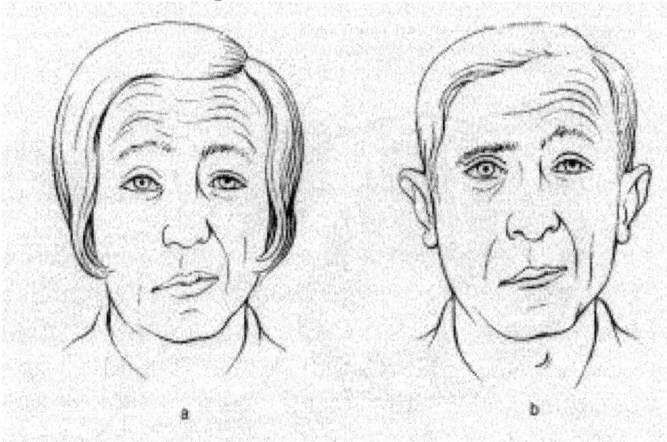

- **ARMS.** Ask the person to raise both arms. See if one arm drifts downward.

- SPEECH. Ask the person to repeat a simple sentence. Check to see if words are slurred and if the sentence is repeated correctly.
- TIME. If a person shows any of these symptoms, time is essential. It is important to get to the hospital as quickly as possible. Call 9-1-1. Act **FAST**.

Clot-Busting Treatment Window Expanded

It is critical for patients with stroke symptoms to get to a hospital as quickly as possible. Patients who are suffering an ischemic stroke may be able to receive a clot-busting drug to dissolve the clot if they reach a hospital within 3 hours of symptom onset.

According to the American Heart Association and the American Stroke Association, this treatment window can be extended to 4.5 hours for patients who:

- Are younger than 80 years old
- Are not having a severe stroke
- Do not have a history of stroke and diabetes
- Do not take oral anticoagulant (blood-thinner) drugs

Drug Approval

In 2011, the Food and Drug Administration (FDA) approved a new anticoagulant drug, rivaroxaban (Xarelto), to prevent stroke and blood clots in patients with atrial fibrillation, a common irregular heart rhythm that is a major cause of stroke. Last year, the FDA approved dabigatran (Pradaxa) for the same purpose. These new anticoagulants may be an alternative to warfarin (Coumadin, generic) for some patients. The FDA is expected to announce in 2012 whether a third new anticoagulant, apixaban (Eliquis), will be approved.

Effects of Stroke

If the stroke occurs toward the back of the brain, for instance, it's likely that some disability involving vision will result. The effects of a stroke depend primarily on the location of the obstruction and the extent of brain tissue affected.

Right Brain:

The effects of a stroke depend on several factors, including the location of the obstruction and how much brain tissue is affected. However, because one side of the brain controls the opposite side of the body, a stroke affecting one side will result in neurological complications on the side of the body it affects. For example, if the stroke occurs in the brain's right side, the left side of the body (and the left side of the face) will be affected, which could produce any or all of the following:

- Paralysis on the left side of the body
- Vision problems
- Quick, inquisitive behavioral style
- Memory loss

Left Brain:

If the stroke occurs in the left side of the brain, the right side of the body will be affected, producing some or all of the following:

- Paralysis on the right side of the body
- Speech/language problems
- Slow, cautious behavioral style
- Memory loss

Effects of a left hemisphere stroke:

The effects of a left hemisphere stroke may include the following:

- right-sided weakness (right hemiparesis) or paralysis (right hemiplegia) and sensory impairment, problems with speech and understanding language (aphasia)
- visual problems, including the inability to see the right visual field of each eye (homonymous hemianopsia)
- impaired ability to do math or to organize, reason, and analyze items
- behavioral changes such as depression, cautiousness, and hesitancy
- impaired ability to read, write, and learn new information
- memory problems

[Summary, Steve Hatch had a Left-Brain Stroke leaving him paralyzed on the right side of his body, trouble speaking, facial weakness, unclear speech and problems with swallowing. He may have had other undiagnosed problems as mentioned above. MJW]

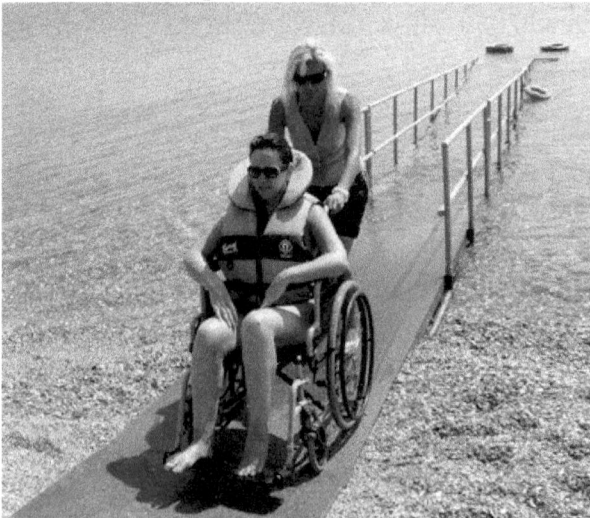

Handicap accessible dock for wheelchair swimmers. Person in chair is well protected with flotation devices.

Affects on Eyesight and the Brain

Symptoms From Blockage in the Carotid Arteries: The carotid arteries stem off of the aorta (the primary artery leading from the heart) and lead up through the neck, around the windpipe, and into the brain. When TIAs or strokes result from clots that form on blockages in the carotid artery, symptoms may occur in either the retina of the eye or the cerebral hemisphere (the large top part of the brain).

Symptoms include:

- When oxygen to the eye is reduced, people describe the visual effect as a shade being pulled down. People may develop poor night vision. About 35% of TIAs are associated with temporary lost vision in one eye. The visual impairment occurs on the same side as the carotid disease.
- When the cerebral hemisphere is affected, a person can have problems with speech and partial and temporary paralysis, drooping eyelid, tingling, and numbness, usually on one side of the body. The stroke victim may be unable to express thoughts verbally or to understand spoken words. If the stroke injuries are on the right side of the brain, the symptoms will develop on the left side of the body and vice versa.
- Uncommonly, patients may have seizures. (What to do during a seizure is included in this book.)

Symptoms From Blockage in the Basilar Artery. The basilar artery is formed at the base of the skull from the vertebral arteries, which run up along the spine and join at the back of the head. When stroke or TIAs originate here, both hemispheres of the brain may be affected so that symptoms occur on both sides of the body. The following symptoms may develop:

- Temporarily dim, gray, blurry, or lost vision, usually in both eyes

- Tingling or numbness in the mouth, cheeks, or gums
- Headache, usually in the back of the head
- Dizziness
- Nausea and vomiting
- Difficulty swallowing
- Weakness in the arms and legs, sometimes causing a sudden fall

Such strokes usually occur in the brain stem, which can have profound effects on breathing, blood pressure, heart rate, and other vital functions, but have no affect on thinking or language.

Speed of Symptom Onset. The speed of symptom onset of a major ischemic stroke may indicate its source:

If the stroke is caused by an embolus (a clot that has traveled to an artery in the brain), the onset is sudden. Headache and seizures can occur within seconds of the blockage.

When thrombosis (a blood clot that has formed within the brain) causes the stroke, the onset usually occurs more gradually, over minutes to hours. On rare occasions it progresses over days to weeks.

Stroke Survivors – Their Stories
Harshada's Story

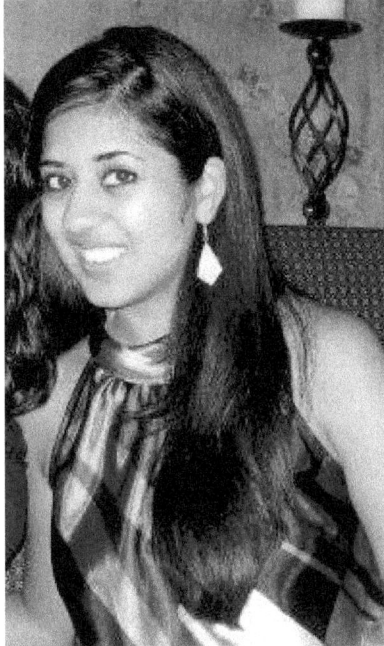

Harshada is a 27-year-old North Carolina native. She graduated from Duke University in 2007 and began medical school at her alma mater immediately thereafter. On November 29, 2008, Harshada suffered a vertebral artery dissection leading to a bilateral brainstem (pontine) stroke. She spent the next nine months completely paralyzed from head to toe. Now, nearly three and a half years later, her life is still a struggle. But through perseverance, the support of family and friends, and her poignant writing, she has begun putting pieces of her life back together.

Have you ever felt invisible? As if your every action and every emotion remained unseen? Has it ever felt like the world was moving and shaking around you, but you were frozen in place, resigned to watching the world unfold without you?

November 29, 2008 -- I woke up in a room I didn't recognize, with no recollection of how I got there. And the kicker: I was completely and painfully alone.

I tried to get up, but my body refused to budge. I tried to cry out, but all that came out of my mouth was silence. Fear coursed through me like a tidal wave, crashing down so forcefully, I swear my heart stopped. After what felt like an eternity, after the terror and curiosity-inspired torture had disseminated my heart into pieces, there was only one thing that could keep me from self-destructing. I saw them. At my bedside were the warm, smiling, familiar faces of my brother and my parents, showing a confidence and peace that felt mystical. For a second there, I felt comforted, like their smiles were shielding me from all those fears and questions that were consuming me. But I couldn't hug them, I couldn't tell them I loved them, I couldn't even smile at them, I could just cry. Cry and cry and cry, and hope that through my silent tears, they could feel my love.

But that fleeting sense of safety only lasted a moment, then it was back to reality, one that was clearly in no rush to go anywhere. Before, when I had a big test coming up in medical school, I would spend hours on Facebook instead of studying, and I would always say, "I'm like totally a waste of space!" Sick twist of fate: now I realized I actually was one. The next few months, and to a slightly lesser extent -- the next few years, I was motionless, speechless, lifeless. I was completely aware of the world around me, but completely unable to interact with it. Some people describe it as being buried alive but I think it feels like something between that and hell.

I couldn't control anything in my world, my life, my happiness, or my future, and for a former control-freak, this was a mental torture I couldn't bear. Everyone would try to be so gentle with me, but it was inevitable that I was beat up everyday. My arm would get stuck under me when they turned me or my foot would get hit during a transfer. But I couldn't do anything about it, except wait and hope someone noticed my pain-stricken, tear-soaked face. If I was so invisible to the world, what the hell was the point in keeping me in this world?

I had to face the fact that I lost a life so full of meaning, and traded it in for one that was painfully meaningless. Would I ever move anything again? Would I ever gain any semblance of my life back? Would my boyfriend still love me? Would anyone still love me? It didn't matter who I was, or what I believed; I couldn't compete with a world that was capable of doing this to me. These thoughts and questions built up inside me and erupted out as a constant stream of tears, all day and all night.

The only battle I could fight was therapy -- I could put my head down and my fears aside, and work harder than I had ever worked before. I couldn't fight with fate but I could certainly work to get the odds in my favor. But besides therapy, what else was I good for? World's oldest blubbering baby? It truly destroyed me was that I wasn't adding anything to the world around me; if anything, I was hurting it and the people around me. I was physically and definitely emotionally really hard to handle. But my family refused to back down, refused to give up on me, refused to let the world keep me invisible. No matter how much I cried or how bleak my future looked, the confidence and peace they showed on that first day, never wavered. They believed in me.

Somewhere, very deep down in my heart, I also had a teeny, tiny belief that I was going to get better, but that belief was hidden beneath all my fears, smothered by all my concerns, and poisoned by the awful things I heard people say. I slowly realized, that alone, yes, I was useless, powerless, *invisible*, but with my family's belief in me, I could be powerful. Fate had silenced us once already with this horrible injury, but we weren't staying quiet anymore. With my ceaseless fighting through therapy, and their relentless push and support, together, we were, and are, a force to be reckoned with. And we won't let fate win.

~ ~

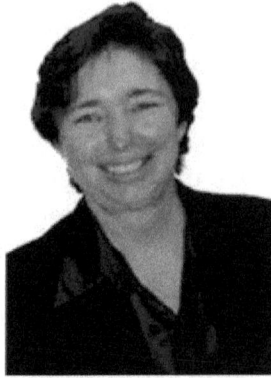

Ruth's Story

Out of the Darkness and Into The Light by Ruth Lycke

Ruth suffered a brain stem bleed and subsequent stroke in November of 2001. Expected to die within the first 24 hours she battled back and lived. Overcoming horrific odds she progressed slowly through the recovery process. As a faithful patient Ruth followed all of her physicians recommendations. 2 1/2 years later she had regained far more than her doctors thought possible. Still 100% disabled she was encouraged by her physicians to accept her condition and be content with what little she had regained.

Faced with seemingly insurmountable odds Ruth refused to be content and was determined to begin a quest to regain all that she had lost. It took years after the stroke for her to discover the answers that would end her suffering with "disabilities" and restore the person she once was.

Follow Ruth as she journeys out of the darkness of the stroke. Experience the tears and joys, frustration and hope, as she uncovers answers in ancient mysteries in a far away land. Join her on the quest that finally brought her into the light.

More about Ruth follows.

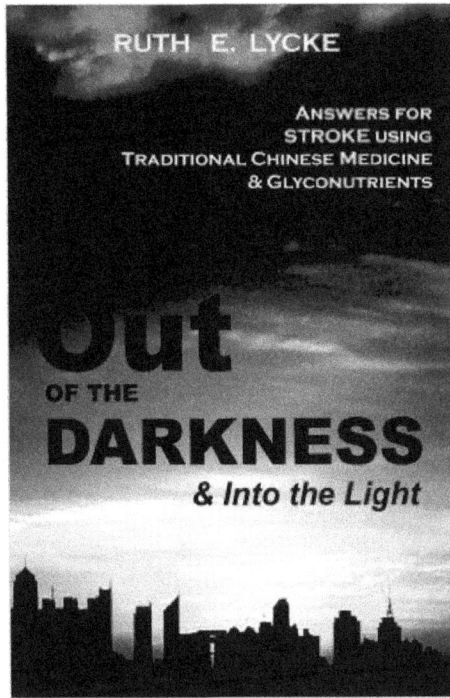

RUTH E. LYCKE

ANSWERS FOR
STROKE USING
TRADITIONAL CHINESE MEDICINE
& GLYCONUTRIENTS

Out
OF THE
DARKNESS
& Into the Light

The following is excerpted from Stroke Connection
Magazine, March/April 2006

"After my stroke, I was a basket case without the basket," said Ruth, mother of three teenagers. It took a trip to China and treatment with that country's non-traditional medicine to get her close to being her old self.

In November 2001, Ruth had an inoperable brain stem hemorrhage. "They thought I would die in the first 24 hours," she said "I actually had two strokes, the brain stem bleed and a secondary stroke. I was in a coma for five days."

When she awoke, she had double vision, no mobility or feeling on the right side of her body, limited left side mobility and no balance. She also had cognitive deficits. "Words were my enemy," she said.

The double vision was profoundly distressing because it affected everything else in her recovery. "Not only did I see two of everything, but everything I looked at bounced. There was constant motion. And any fatigue would prevent me from thinking linearly. I repeated myself a lot, which challenged my husband Steve and our three kids, who were between the ages of 9 and 13 at that time."

By two years post-stroke, she had made a remarkable recovery, but her life and her body were not where she wanted them. "I still had double vision and difficulty walking. I was incontinent. I didn't get out very much, and when I did, it was difficult. I became more or less a shut-in."

There was no stroke support group in her hometown of Marshalltown, Iowa, so she started one with the help of the American Stroke Association.

"My doctors told me to be content with what had returned," she said. "But nothing worked right, so I wasn't content."

They had hosted foreign exchange students for several years, and during this period they hosted two girls from China. Ruth learned about Chinese medicine from them, and they used their Chinese language skills to search the Internet for information on stroke and traditional medicine. That's how she found the First Teaching Hospital and University of Traditional Chinese Medicine in Tianjin, China.

After forwarding her medical records to the hospital, she talked to a doctor. "He asked me, 'What do you want me to do for you?' I had never had a doctor ask me that question before. So I gave him my list: normal vision, restored balance, feeling on my right side, improved walking and fine motor movement on my right side. Then he said, 'We can fix you.' I couldn't believe it, so I asked him to repeat it."

Ruth flew to China alone, a long trek for someone with her deficits. Once there, she was escorted by the families of her exchange students until she reached the hospital. "I arrived at 10 in the morning, and by 2 o'clock I was already in therapy," she said. "Their therapy is very intense. I had acupuncture twice a day, involving anywhere from 40 to 100 needles – from the tip of my head to my toes on both sides. By the way, the needles don't hurt. They're very thin.

"I also had herbal soaks on my right foot and arm. Then there was 40 to 60 minutes of intense massage, which is done by a doctor. I was busy from early morning to late at night every day."

Ruth had tried acupuncture in the United States with limited results, but "after my first treatment in China, my little finger felt normal for the first time since the stroke. Within 10 days I regained some degree of feeling in my entire right side. Things would go from no feeling, to intense pain, to weighty feeling, to normal.

"When feeling began to return, I was like a kid in a candy shop," said Ruth. "I would reach out and touch the wall, feel the bumps or the crack where the paint came together. It was remarkable to me."

Although the hospital treats many Europeans, she was its first American patient, so Ruth received lots of attention. "Probably once a week I went to dinner with a doctor. In fact, it wasn't unusual to have dinner with two or three doctors."

The food was an important part of the experience, and one of the most impressive. "All the food was farm fresh. I had an egg or rice soup for breakfast, and then ordered traditional Chinese food for the evening meal from an English menu. The food was very good."

Ruth's treatment cost about $4,000 a month, including meals and a comfortable room. After two months, she had made enough progress that she extended her stay for five months, "to get everything fixed, especially my vision." She considers the $20,000 a bargain for the results produced.

Her experience was good enough that she returned to Tianjin last summer, accompanying two American stroke survivors for treatment. She has four trips planned for 2006.

"I no longer suffer from bouncing double vision, even when I'm tired," Ruth said. "I can jump around on the basketball court with my 14-year-old daughter Elizabeth, who is also very excited that I can walk now, so I can take her to the mall. My balance is back, and the fine motor stuff is returning. I can use the remote control now, and scissors. I can walk without difficulty. I have feeling in my face. Words are my friend again. I wrote a book about my experience, and it's been published. Everything on my list was done. They pretty much gave me my life back."

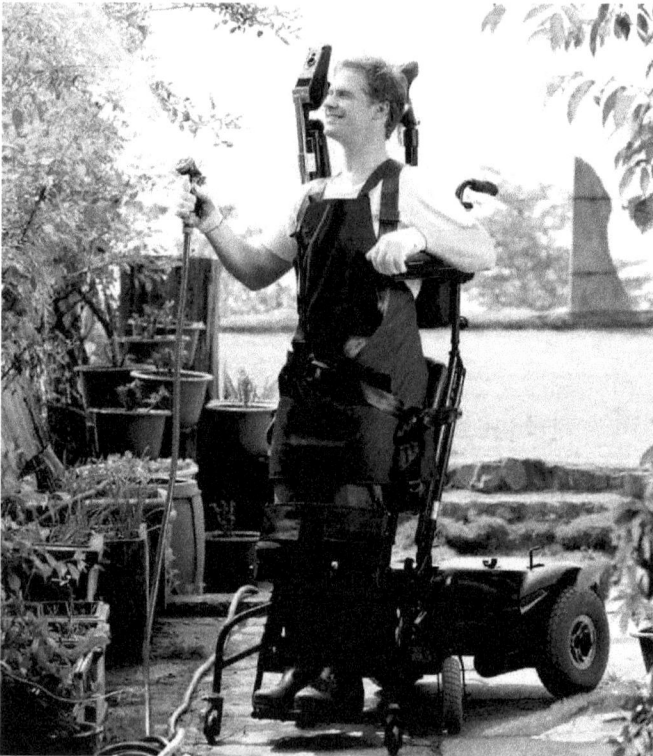

↳Young paralyzed man using stand-up electric wheelchair for his employment in a garden center. He is currently spraying plants with a garden hose.

Stroke Rehabilitation by Mayo Clinic
What to expect as you recover

Stroke rehabilitation (stroke rehab) is an important part of recovery after stroke. Find out what's involved in stroke rehabilitation.

The goal of a stroke rehabilitation program is to help you relearn skills you lost when stroke affected part of your brain. Stroke rehabilitation can help you regain independence and improve your quality of life.

The severity of stroke complications and each person's ability to recover lost abilities varies widely. Researchers have found that the central nervous system is adaptive and can recover some functions. They also have found that it's necessary to keep practicing regained skills.

What's involved in stroke rehabilitation?

There are numerous approaches to stroke rehabilitation, some of which are still in the early stages of development. Behavioral performance in any area, such as sensory motor and cognitive function, is most likely to improve when motor activity is willful, repetitive and task specific.

Stroke rehabilitation may include some or all of the following activities, depending on the part of the body or type of ability affected.

Physical activities:
- **Strengthening motor skills** involves using exercises to help improve your muscle strength and coordination, including therapy to help with swallowing.
- **Mobility training** may include learning to use walking aids, such as a walker or canes, or a plastic brace (orthosis) to stabilize and assist ankle strength to help support your body's weight while you relearn how to walk.

- **Constraint-induced therapy,** also known as forced-use therapy, involves restricting use of an unaffected limb while you practice moving the affected limb to help improve its function.

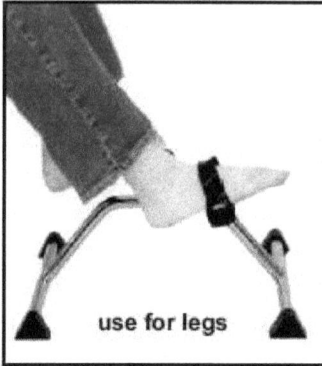

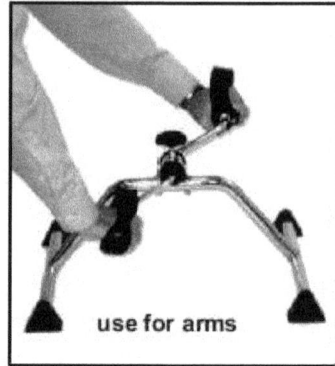

use for legs

use for arms

- **Range-of-motion therapy** uses exercises and other treatments to help lessen muscle tension (spasticity) and regain range of motion. Sometimes medication can help as well.

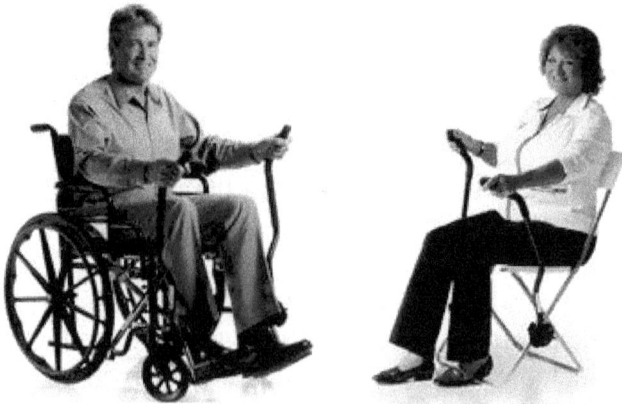

Portable Exercise bars for arm movement can be used while seated.

See "Inventions and Aids for Stroke Victims" for additional pictures of manually operated, motorized, and other inventions for partially paralyzed people.

Technology-assisted physical activities:

- **Functional electrical stimulation** involves using electricity to stimulate weakened muscles, causing them to contract. This may help with muscle re-education.
- **Robotic technology** uses robotic devices to assist impaired limbs with performing repetitive motions, helping them regain strength and function. A recent large study showed no clear advantage to using robotic technology to improve motor recovery after stroke.
- **Wireless technology,** such as a simple activity monitor, is being evaluated for its benefit in increasing post-stroke activity.
- **Virtual reality,** such as the use of video games, is an emerging, computer-based therapy that involves interacting with a simulated, real-time environment.
- **Noninvasive brain stimulation.** Techniques such as transcranial magnetic stimulation (TMS) have been used to help improve a variety of motor skills.

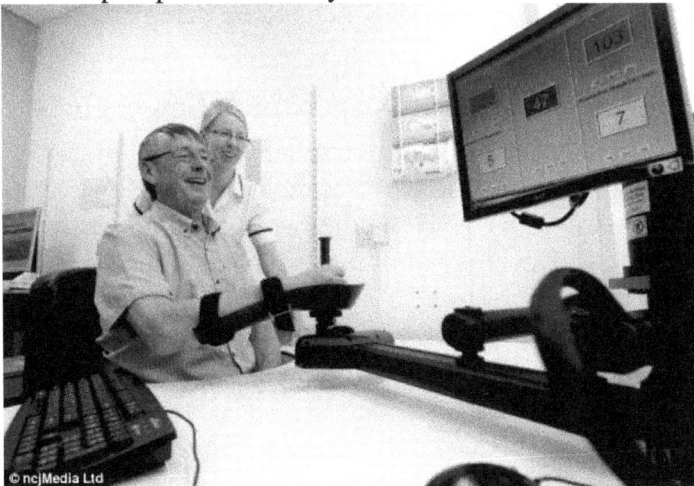

↳Man using robotics to interact with his paralyzed arm. The machine starts the movement and assists when sensing movement from the man's arm.

Cognitive and Emotional Activities:

- **Therapy for communication disorders** can help you regain lost abilities in speaking, listening, writing and comprehension.
- **Psychological evaluation and treatment** may involve testing your cognitive skills and emotional adjustment, counseling with a mental health professional, or participating in support groups.
- **Medications** are sometimes used to treat depression in people who have had a stroke. Drugs that affect movement are also used.

Experimental therapies:

- **Biological therapies,** such as stem cells, are being investigated, but should only be used as part of a clinical trial.
- **Alternative medicine** treatments, such as massage, herbal therapy and acupuncture, are being evaluated.

When should stroke rehabilitation begin?

The sooner you begin stroke rehabilitation, the more likely you are to regain lost abilities and skills. However, your doctors' first priority is to stabilize your medical condition and control life-threatening conditions. They also take measures to prevent another stroke and limit any stroke-related complications.

It's common for stroke rehabilitation to start as soon as 24 to 48 hours after your stroke, during your acute hospital stay. If your medical problems continue for longer, your doctors may wait to begin your rehabilitation.

How long does stroke rehabilitation last?

The duration of your stroke rehabilitation depends on the severity of your stroke and related complications. Although some stroke survivors recover quickly, most need some form of stroke rehabilitation long term, possibly months or years after their stroke.

Your stroke rehabilitation plan will change during your recovery as you relearn skills and your needs change. With ongoing practice, you can continue to make gains over time.

The length of each stroke rehabilitation therapy session varies depending on your recovery, severity of your symptoms and responsiveness to therapy.

Where does stroke rehabilitation take place?

You'll probably begin stroke rehabilitation while you're still in the hospital. Before you leave, you and your family will work with hospital social workers and your care team to determine the best rehabilitation setting depending on your needs, what insurance will cover, and what is most convenient for you and your family. These options include:

- **Inpatient rehabilitation units.** These facilities are either freestanding or part of a larger hospital or clinic. You may stay at the facility for several weeks as part of an intensive rehabilitation program.
- **Outpatient units.** These facilities are often part of a hospital or clinic. You may spend several hours a day at the unit, but return home each night.
- **Skilled nursing facilities.** The type of care available at a nursing facility — sometimes referred to as a nursing home — varies. Some facilities specialize in rehabilitation, while others offer less-intense therapy options.
- **Home-based programs.** Having your therapy at home allows greater flexibility than other options. One drawback is you likely won't have access to specialized

rehabilitation equipment. In addition, insurance strictly controls who qualifies for home-based therapy.

Talk to your doctor and family about the best option for you.

Who participates in your stroke rehabilitation team?

Stroke rehabilitation involves a variety of specialists. Some specialists help with physical needs, including:

- **Physicians** include your primary care doctor as well as specialists in physical medicine and rehabilitation (physiatrists) and neurologists. They help guide your care and prevent complications. They also help you to gain and maintain healthy lifestyle behaviors to avoid another stroke.
- **Rehabilitation nurses** specialize in caring for people with limitations to activities. They help incorporate skills learned in physical, occupational and speech therapy into your daily routines. They also can offer options for managing bowel and bladder complications of stroke.
- **Physical therapists** help you relearn movements such as walking and keeping your balance.
- **Occupational therapists** help you relearn functional hand and arm use for daily skills, such as bathing, tying your shoes or buttoning your shirt. They can also address safety issues in your home, and help with cognitive organizational tasks.

Other specialists focus on cognitive, emotional and vocational skills, including:

- **Speech and language pathologists** help improve your language skills and ability to swallow. They may also teach you how to use compensation tools to address memory, thinking and communication problems.

- **Dietitians** assist you with creating healthy menus, including heart-healthy, low-fat and low-salt foods.
- **Social workers** help connect you to financial resources, as well as help you plan for new living arrangements, if necessary, and identify community resources.
- **Psychologists** assess your thinking skills and help address your mental and emotional health concerns.
- **Therapeutic recreation specialists** help you resume activities and roles you enjoyed before your stroke, including hobbies and community participation.
- **Vocational counselors** help you address return-to-work issues if this is a goal. They can provide information about the Americans with Disabilities Act (ADA) to help with workplace accommodations, if needed.

How to help when a loved has had a stroke.

Stroke is a complicated picture because it may affect your loved one's personality, their ability to pay attention and remember, or the way they express emotions. Recovering from a stroke often isn't a matter of days or week, it can take months, and in some cases, even years. To help your loved one cope and recover from a stroke, try these tips:

- Understand there may be cognitive, personality, language, communication and emotional changes.
- Know that your loved one may become indifferent to family members if their emotional expression has been altered.
- Take them to rehab and go with them to all doctor's appointments. Take notes as the physician talks and ask questions he may have forgotten to ask. Your loved one may be too stressed out to listen and understand, or they may have suffered memory problems that interfere with effective communicating.

- Learn to use available local resources such as nurses' aides, home healthcare aides, church workers and senior daycare programs.
- If you can no longer care for your loved one at home, don't feel guilty about looking into outside options like nursing homes.
- Remember that with a severe stroke, you're not looking at a sprint but a marathon. Don't take on too much too soon or wear yourself out early on. Let other people help you, and make sure to replenish yourself to prevent caregiver burnout.

What affects the outcome of stroke rehabilitation?

Because stroke recovery varies from person to person, it's hard to predict how many abilities you might recover and how soon. In general, successful stroke rehabilitation depends on:

- **Physical factors,** including the severity of your stroke in terms of both cognitive and physical effects
- **Emotional factors,** such as your motivation and mood, and your ability to stick with rehabilitation activities outside of therapy sessions
- **Social factors,** such as the support of <u>friends</u> and family *[Steve Hatch was not allowed by the medical profession to have his 12-year companion be involved in his rehab and care because she was not related. MJW]*
- **Therapeutic factors,** including an early start to your rehabilitation and the skill of your stroke rehabilitation team

Generally the rate of recovery is greatest in the acute and post-acute periods — weeks and months after a stroke. However, there is evidence that performance can improve well into the chronic phase, or years later.

Stroke rehabilitation takes time

Recovering from a stroke can be a long and sometimes frustrating experience. It's normal to face difficulties along the way. Dedication and willingness to work toward improvement will help you gain the most benefit.

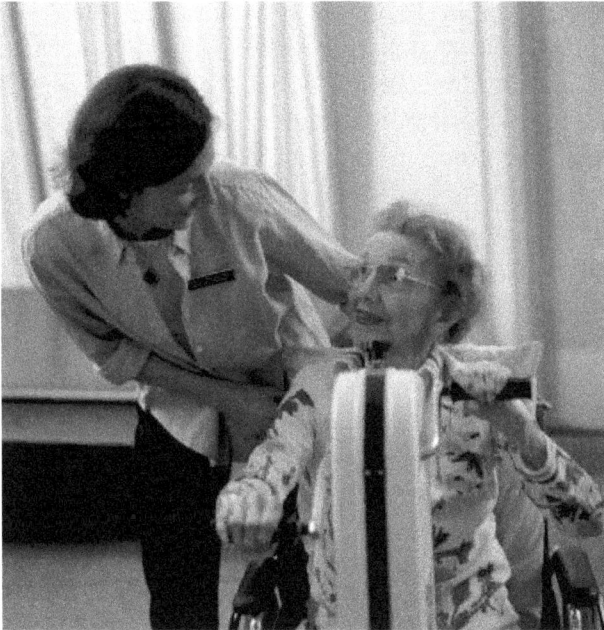

Therapist working with lady using hand-motion equipment. The active arm movement also stimulates the paralyzed arm/hand.

Stroke Recovery – An Explanation

Each person has a different recovery time and need for long-term care.

Where to Live After A Stroke

Most patients will need stroke rehabilitation (rehab) to help them recover after they leave the hospital. Stroke rehab will help you regain the ability to care for yourself. Most types of therapy can be done in the home where you live. Those who are able to go back home might also attend a special clinic or have someone come to their home. Your location also depends on your ability to take care of yourself and how much help there will be at home

Another factor will be whether the home is a safe place -- for example, stairs in the home might not be safe for a stroke patient who has trouble walking

People who are not able to care for themselves at home after a stroke may have therapy in a special part of a hospital or in a nursing or rehabilitation center. Other options could be a boarding home or convalescent home to have a safe environment.

For people who are cared for at home changes may be needed to stay safe from falls in the home and bathroom, prevent wandering, and make the home easier to use. The bed and bathroom should be easy to reach. Items such as throw rugs that may cause a fall should be removed.

A number of devices can help with activities such as cooking or eating, bathing or showering, moving around the home or elsewhere, dressing and grooming, writing and using a computer, and many more activities

Family counseling may help you cope with the changes needed for home care. Visiting nurses or aides, volunteer services, homemakers, adult protective services, adult day care, and other community resources (such as a local Department of Aging) may be helpful.

Legal advice may be needed. Advance directives, power of attorney, and other legal actions may make it easier to make decisions about care.

Author's Note: *[Steve Hatch had a shared home to go to. I am an experienced care-giver and with the help of Home Health Care, I was ready to give him the therapy and care he needed. He had the best insurance and personal assets to get the best equipment and therapists. But I was NOT allowed to help with his care because I was not related to him. Our 12-year companionship did not matter to the medical profession.*

He had not spoken to his older brother for over 20 years. Yet the brother was given 100% control over Steve's care and future even though the laws say NO ONE has the legal right to make decisions on Steve's life except Steve.

Steven Lee Hatch was able to answer "yes" or "no" to questions, there was nothing wrong with his mind. HE alone had the authority to make decisions on his care – except no one asked him and he was taken out of skilled, curative care and put into hospice against his will. Thirteen days later he was dead.. MJW]

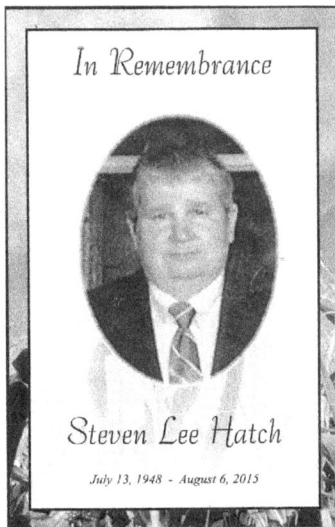

In Remembrance

Steven Lee Hatch

July 13, 1948 - August 6, 2015

Speaking and Communicating

After a stroke, some people may have problems finding a word or being able to speak more than one word or phrase at a time. Or, they may have trouble speaking at all which is called aphasia.

People who have had a stroke may be able to put many words together, but they may not make sense. Patients may not know that what they are saying is not easy to understand. They may get frustrated when they realize other people cannot understand them.

A stroke can also damage the muscles that help you speak. As a result, these muscles do not move the right way when you try to speak. It can take up to 2 years to recover speech. Not everyone will fully recover. A speech and language therapist can work with you and your family or caregivers.

There are other ways you can communicate.

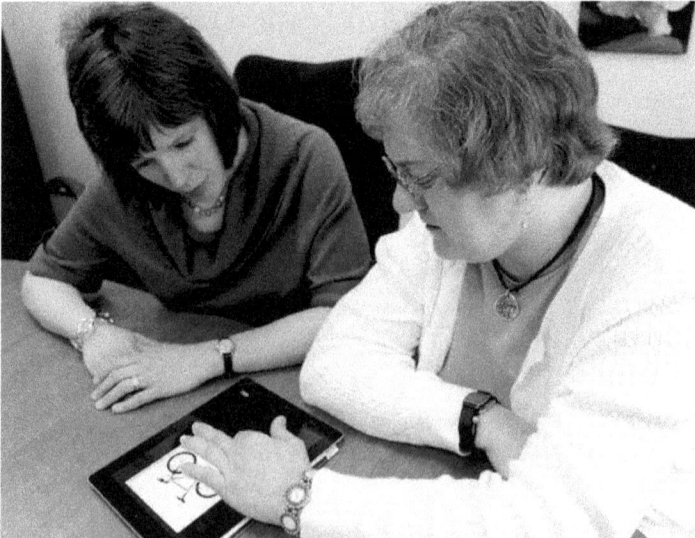

Cathy Dykeman recognizes the striped animal shown on the virtual flash card in the Name That! application on her tablet. She carefully spells out the word on the brown office table at the University of Northern Iowa's speech communications center with her finger.

Z ... E ... B ...

Despite successfully spelling it, she cannot say it. The area of her brain that controls speech isn't the same since she suffered a stroke in 1998. She stumbles on the word. She gives up.

"Zebra," the voice on the app tells her after she pushes a button.

The 51-year-old Waterloo resident flashes a smile. "I knew that one," she says.

Dykeman has helped test an app developed by Northern Iowa professor and speech pathologist Angie Burda that helps victims of strokes exercise the speech part of the brain as they recover. The application is part of a growing number of technology-related products making life easier for people with speech disabilities, including victims of strokes and those who stutter.

"After people have a stroke, they have difficulty speaking," Burda said. "They know they are looking at a cup or a pencil. But they just can't access that information."

With the app, patients can test the speech parts of their brain at home, instead of having to wait for appointments with a speech therapist.

Dykeman has met with a therapist in an attempt to build her vocabulary since a night in 1998 that changed her life, when she woke up slurring her speech.

As a human resources manager in Minneapolis, Dykeman lived comfortably with her two kittens. When she woke in a daze. She couldn't form any words and garbled her speech.

When she called 911, the dispatcher thought she was drunk.

"I was so mad because I didn't know who I was," she said. "I didn't know what to do." Doctors told her she had suffered a stroke.

It often comes with debilitating effects, and Dykeman's stroke included the disorder known as aphasia, which results from damage to the language parts of the brain.

She also lost the ability to use the right side of her body. When doctors told her, she immediately wondered how she would be able to continue working.

"I can't work there anymore, I can't do it," she thought to herself.

She moved in with her mother, who lives in Waterloo, and soon found speech pathologist Angie Burda.

Speech therapists use semantic feature analysis to help stroke victims regain their speech processes. The method puts information in front of people that leads to connections between objects and actions to help them form words.

For example, a therapist could put a picture of a rocking chair in front of a patient and ask what they are used for. The patient will try to make connections and say the word "sit."

Burda wanted to find a way to put that into a mobile application. Thanks to a Northern Iowa program that connects professors from different parts of the school, she found someone to build it in 2011.

"So many people now have smartphones and tablets," she said. "We have 80-year-olds who have iPads. You are providing them the opportunity to improve."

Students from both the computer science and communication sciences and disorders departments developed the application, with Stephen Hughes, the AppsLab manager at the John Pappajohn Entrepreneurial Center at UNI, leading its development.

It joins a growing market of speech therapy applications available in Apple's App Store. The goal is to sell the product to other speech therapists for use with patients, but Name That! remains available for anyone to download for $4.99.

Once Hughes developed a working version of the app, he and Burda sought a patient willing to experiment with it.

That led to one of Burda's more dedicated patients, Cathy Dykeman, in late 2012. Dykeman had been working with Angie Burda since 2000. But as much as Burda's guidance helps Dykeman's recovery, the two only meet for two 50-minute sessions a week.

"Usually, pathologists and their patients are only together for a short period of time," Burda said. "They can go home, use this app, and hopefully it leads to improved communication down the road."

Dykeman said she's seen improvement since she started testing the app. Still, she's frustrated when words she has known all her life are no longer easily accessible.

She grits her teeth when asked what it feels like to not be able to access the parts of her brain she needs to find those words.

"It makes me so mad," she said. "I can't speak sometimes. That's what I really don't understand — why I can't speak."

Dykeman has accepted that her full-time job is recovering. A filing job at a Waterloo medical office helped her feel better about herself.

That part of recovery is crucial because Dykeman sometimes feels the hurtful words she hears from cashiers or others who wonder what is wrong with her.

"They say, 'What, are you dumb or weird?" she said. "But I tell them I had a stroke, and they say 'Oh, OK."

Burda said she enjoys watching patients slowly move toward a semblance of their former life. She hopes the application will supplement therapy sessions enough to help reach that goal.

"The idea has always been to augment the relationship between patient and therapist," she said. "This is a long-term process. The application is not going to fix it on its own."

Thinking and Memory

After a stroke, people may have:

- Changes in their ability to think or reason
- Changes in behavior
- Memory problems
- Poor judgment

These problems increase the need for safety precautions.

Depression after a stroke is common. It can start soon afterward or may not begin for up to 2 years after the stroke. Treatments for depression include increased social activity, more visits in the home or going to an adult day care center for activities. The person may need medicines for depression and visits to a therapist or counselor.

Muscle, Joint and Nerve Problems

Moving around and doing normal daily tasks such as dressing and feeding may be harder after a stroke. Muscles on one side of the body may be weaker or may not move at all. This may involve only part of the arm or leg, or the whole side of the body. Also muscles on the weak side of the body may be very tight. A hand splint may be applied while you are in the hospital to reduce risk of contractures -- a condition in which fingers get "stuck" in a bent position (more on that later.)

Different joints in the body may become hard to move. The shoulder and other joints may dislocate since the patient is unable to tighten their muscles to keep the arm-joint from separating. Many of these problems can cause pain after a stroke. Pain may also occur from changes in the brain itself. You may use pain medicines, but check with your health care provider first. People who have pain due to tight muscles may get medicines that help with muscle spasms.

Physical therapists, occupational therapists, and rehabilitation doctors will help you relearn how to:

- Dress, groom, and eat
- Bathe, shower, and use the toilet
- Use canes, walkers, wheelchairs, and other devices to stay as mobile as possible

- Possibly return to work
- Keep all of the muscles as strong as possible and stay as physically active as possible, even if you cannot walk
- Manage muscle spasms or tightness with stretching exercises and braces that fit around the ankle, elbow, shoulder, and other joints

Bladder and Bowel Care

A stroke can lead to problems with bladder or bowel control. These problems may be caused by damage to part of the brain that helps the bowels and bladder work smoothly. You may not notice the need to go to the bathroom or have a problem getting to the toilet in time

Other symptoms may include loss of bowel control, diarrhea (loose bowel movements), or constipation (hard bowel movements), loss of bladder control, feeling the need to urinate often, or problems emptying the bladder.

Certain medicines your doctor may prescribe may help with bladder control. You may need a referral to a bladder or bowel specialist. Sometimes, a bladder or bowel schedule will help. It can also help to place a commode chair close to where you sit most of the day. Some people need a permanent urinary catheter to drain urine from their body.

To prevent skin or pressure sores clean up after incontinence, change position often and know how to move in a bed, chair, or wheelchair. Make sure the wheelchair fits correctly and gives you the support for your head and your weak side.

Have family members or other caregivers learn how to watch out for skin sores as you may not have feeling in the areas where pressure sores have developed.

Swallowing and Eating After A Stroke

Swallowing problems may be cause by damage to the nerves that help you swallow. Symptoms of swallowing problems are:

- Coughing or choking, either during or after eating
- Gurgling sounds from the throat during or after eating
- Throat clearing after drinking or swallowing
- Slow chewing or eating
- Coughing food back up after eating
- Hiccups after swallowing
- Chest discomfort during or after swallowing

A speech therapist can help with swallowing and eating problems after a stroke. Diet changes, such as thickening liquids or eating pureed foods, may be needed. Some people will need a permanent a gastric feeding tube (G-tube) which is inserted through a small incision in the abdomen into the stomach and is used for long-term enteral nutrition. One type is the percutaneous endoscopic gastrostomy (PEG) tube which is placed endoscopically.

Some people do not take in enough calories after a stroke. High-calorie foods or food supplements that also contain vitamins or minerals can prevent weight loss and keep you healthy.

It is normal to feel angry, anxious or depressed after a stroke. You may feel worried about work, money and relationships, and the tiredness caused by stroke can make things worse.

Rehabilitation is about getting back to normal life and living as independent a life as possible. It involves taking an active approach to ensure that your life goes on. This can mean learning new skills or relearning old ones. It may involve adapting to new limitations and post-stroke conditions. Or it can mean finding new social, emotional, and practical support to live your best life post-stroke.

You may find new hobbies and activities to do that you never had time to pursue before. You may connect with other people with the same or different disabilities which you can help them to improve their outlook while boosting your own progress and attitude and perspective.

With good care and rehabilitation, there is life after stroke.

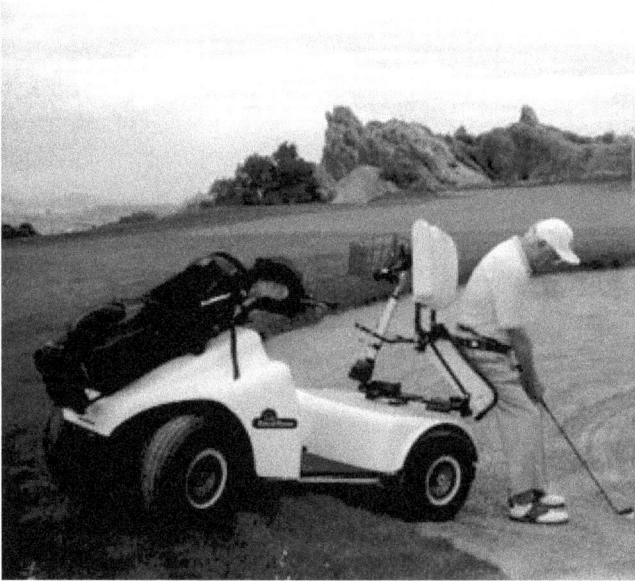

Man golfing with cart supported by swivel seat.

Other Recovery Information

Early recovery

There's still so much we don't know about how the brain compensates for the damage caused by stroke. In some cases, the brain cells may be only temporarily damaged, not killed, and may resume functioning over time. In other cases, the brain can reorganize its own functioning. Every once in a while, a region of the brain "takes over" for a region damaged by the stroke. Stroke survivors sometimes experience remarkable and unanticipated recoveries that can't be explained. General recovery guidelines show:

> - 10% of stroke survivors recover almost completely
> - 25% recover with minor impairments
> - 40% experience moderate to severe impairments requiring special care
> - 10% require care in a nursing home or other long-term care facility
> - 15% die shortly after the stroke

Your recovery team

To help you meet your stroke recovery goals, your rehab program will be planned by a team of professionals. This team may include some of the following:

- **Physiatrist.** Specializes in rehabilitation following injuries, accidents or illness
- **Neurologist.** Specializes in the prevention, diagnosis and treatment of stroke and other diseases of the brain and spinal cord
- **Rehabilitation Nurse.** Specializes in helping people with disabilities; helps survivors manage health problems that affect stroke (diabetes, high blood pressure) and adjust to life after stroke

- **Physical Therapist** (PT). Helps stroke survivors with problems in moving and balance; suggests exercises to strengthen muscles for walking, standing and other activities
- **Occupational Therapist** (OT). Helps stroke survivors learn strategies to manage daily activities such as eating, bathing, dressing, writing or cooking
- **Speech-Language Pathologists** (SLP). Helps stroke survivors re-learn language skills (talking, reading and writing); shares strategies to help with swallowing problems
- **Dietician**. Teaches survivors about healthy eating and special diets (low salt, low fat, low calorie)
- **Social Worker**. Helps survivors make decisions about rehab programs, living arrangements, insurance, and support services in the home
- **Neuropsychologist**. Diagnoses and treats survivors who may be facing changes in thinking, memory, and behavior after stroke
- **Case Manager.** Helps survivors facilitate follow-up to acute care, coordinate care from multiple providers, and link to local services
- **Recreation Therapist**. Helps stroke survivors learn strategies to improve the thinking and movement skills needed to join in recreational activities

(Steve Hatch did not receive any of the above "Recovery Team" services. He was giving minimal care, no mental stimulation, and his 12-year companion was not included in any discussion for his future plans. MJW)

A primary concern immediately after stroke for patients, their relatives, and their caregivers is the prospect for recovery. To address this concern and to aid in clinical management, individual predictions of recovery are needed; information about the "average" recovery pattern may have little relevance to an individual clinician or the patient. Prognostic studies of outcome after stroke have tended to concentrate on predicting outcome at a specific time point such as 6 months after stroke. This type of prediction does not aid clinical decisions about whether to continue an intervention such as a rehabilitation program or the identification of causes of failure to recover. The patient's rate of recovery also has important implications for costs of care, especially the length of hospital stay.

Stroke Recovery and Arm Rehab
Important Questions

1) **What caused my stroke?** Eighty percent of all strokes occur when blood flow to the brain is suddenly cut off -- usually by a blood clot or some other obstruction. This is called an ischemic stroke. A hemorrhagic stroke occurs when a blood vessel ruptures in the brain. Knowing the type of stroke you had can help your doctor determine the underlying cause. For example, an ischemic stroke may be caused by a blocked artery due to the buildup of plaque -- a mixture of cholesterol and other lipids, or blood fats. People with atherosclerosis, or hardening of the arteries from plaque buildup, are more at risk for this type of stroke. High blood pressure is a common culprit in hemorrhagic stroke. Both of these conditions increase the risk of stroke, and managing them can help prevent a second stroke.

2) **Am I at risk for a second stroke?** The overall risk of a second stroke is highest right after a stroke. Three percent of survivors have a second stroke in the first 30 days, and one-third will have another within two years. It's vital to talk with your doctor to understand your specific risk factors and develop a plan to minimize them. High blood pressure is the biggest risk factor for stroke. Having heart disease, high blood cholesterol, or diabetes also puts you at

risk. Lifestyle factors that put you at risk include smoking cigarettes, obesity, physical inactivity, heavy alcohol consumption, and illicit drug use.

3) **What is the stroke recovery process?** Although your stroke rehabilitation program will be tailored to your specific needs, most people follow a similar path. You'll begin to do assisted exercises in the hospital once your medical condition has stabilized. From there, you may go to an in-patient rehab facility where you will receive intensive therapy to help you become more independent. Once you are able to return home, you may receive outpatient therapy or home therapy. Formal rehabilitation takes place for about three to six months. But stroke patients who continue to practice the skills they learned in rehabilitation continue to see progress long after a stroke has occurred.

4) **How long will my recovery from stroke take?** Stroke recovery is different for every patient. Although some people with a mild stroke recover quickly, for most stroke survivors, recovery is a lifelong process. While the biggest gains will be made in the first three months after a stroke, patients can continue to recover ... even years later. The key is to get into a daily pattern of exercise.

5) **Am I at risk for depression after a stroke?** Becoming depressed after a stroke is very common. So ask your doctor about the symptoms of depression so that you and your caregivers know what to look for. Post-stroke depression is thought to be caused in part by biochemical changes in the brain. It's also a completely normal reaction to the losses caused by a stroke. Whatever the reason, treatment is essential. Fortunately, depression can be effectively treated with medication and/or counseling.

6) **What medications will I be taking and do they have any side effects?** Strokes are most often caused by blood clots, so your doctor will probably prescribe anticoagulant or

antiplatelet medication, commonly known as blood thinners, to help prevent future strokes.

You may also need to take medications to help lower high blood pressure or high cholesterol, treat a heart condition, or manage diabetes. *[Steve Hatch was already on medications for high blood pressure, high cholesterol, a defective heart valve, and to manage diabetes yet when he was forced into "hospice and unskilled care" without his permission, his prior medications were replaced with palliative medications (sedatives and morphin.) and he died 13 days later. MJW]*

Be sure to talk with your doctor about your medications so that you understand why you are taking them. Ask about potential side effects and possible food and medicine interactions. To help you keep track, you or your caregiver should write down the name and dose of all your medications, including when and how to take them.

Speech Skills

Strokes can cause a language impairment called aphasia. People with this condition have trouble speaking in general or have specific problems, such as not using the right words or not speaking in full sentences. Strokes can also prevent you from speaking normally if they damage the muscles that control speech. Speech and language therapists can help you try to speak coherently and clearly. If the damage is too severe, they can teach you other ways to communicate.

Cognitive Skills

Strokes can impair your thinking and reasoning abilities, lead to poor judgment, and cause memory problems. They can also cause behavioral changes. You may have once been outgoing and exuberant, but are now shy and withdrawn, or vice versa. In some cases, stroke survivors are more prone to risk-taking behaviors due to not understanding the consequences of their actions or having fewer inhibitions.

The medical experts who help you rehabilitate can also affect how well you recover. The more skilled they are, the better your recovery will be. Your family members and friends can also help improve your outlook by providing encouragement and support. You can increase your chances of successfully recovering by practicing your rehabilitation exercises on a regular basis.

Recovery Statistics

The National Stroke Association states that 10 percent of people who have had a stroke make a full recovery, 25 percent have only minor complications, and 40 percent end up needing special care for moderate to severe problems. Only 10 percent require long-term care in a nursing home or other facility.

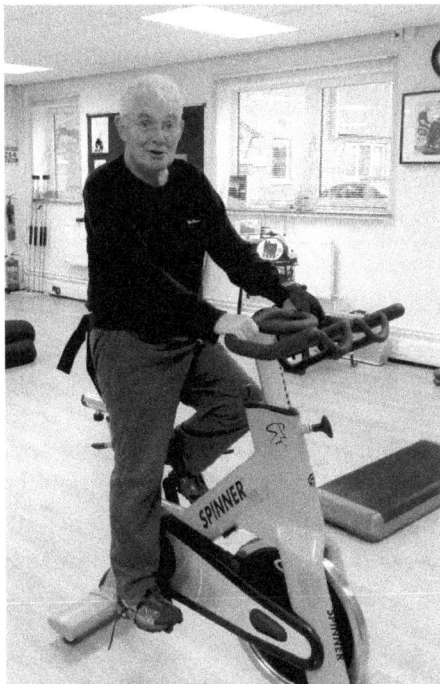

🔖Man exercising in the rehab center on stationary bike.

Technical Stroke Descriptions

Hemorrhagic Stroke

There are two main types of stroke: hemorrhagic and ischemic. A hemorrhagic stroke occurs when blood vessels in the brain rupture, causing blood to accumulate in the surrounding brain tissue. This causes pressure on the brain, which can be problematic. The rupture can also leave part of the brain deprived of blood and oxygen. Only 13 percent of strokes are hemorrhagic, according to the American Stroke Association.

Ischemic Stroke

The majority of strokes are ischemic. An ischemic stroke results from a clot that blocks blood flow to a particular region of the brain. The clot may be a cerebral thrombosis, meaning it forms at the site of the blockage in the brain. Alternatively, the clot may be a cerebral embolism, which means it forms elsewhere in the body and moves into the brain, causing a stroke.

Severity of Strokes

Strokes can range from minor and almost unnoticeable to massive and fatal. The National Institutes of Health created a tool used by health professionals to measure the severity of a stroke. It uses a number score to rate the severity of the symptoms, and therefore the severity of the stroke.

Symptoms measured by the scale include consciousness, eye movement, facial palsy, arm and leg mobility, sensation, language, and speech. Points on the scale range from zero to 42, with a rating from 21 to 42 indicating a severe, or massive, stroke.

Hemorrhagic Stroke Symptoms

A hemorrhagic stroke may occur within the brain or on the surface of the brain. Symptoms of the former include a severe headache, confusion, nausea, vomiting, and seizures. The more severe these symptoms, the more massive the stroke is.

If the stroke occurs on the surface of the brain, symptoms are slightly different. These symptoms may include headache, vomiting, neck stiffness, loss of vision, or in severe cases, rigidity and coma. Symptoms of hemorrhagic strokes begin suddenly, but often worsen over the course of a few hours.

Ischemic Stroke Symptoms

An ischemic stroke often begins with a sudden severe headache, dizziness and loss of balance or coordination, blurred vision, numbness and weakness in one side of the face and body, sudden confusion, and difficulty talking. The severity of symptoms depends how massive the stroke is.

Hemorrhagic Stroke Treatment

In order to slow the bleeding caused by a hemorrhagic stroke, emergency caregivers may give a patient medications to lower blood pressure. If the patient has been on blood thinners, he or she may be given drugs to counteract them, as these medications worsen bleeding.

A patient experiencing a hemorrhagic stroke may need emergency surgery, depending on the severity of the bleeding. This is done to repair the broken blood vessel and to remove excess blood that may be putting dangerous pressure on the brain.

Ischemic Stroke Treatment

Emergency care for a stroke must be administered as soon as possible. The promptness of treatment is important for recovery. The sooner treatment can be given, the better the odds of survival and recovery. For an ischemic stroke, emergency care involves targeting and dissolving the clot. Clot-busting drugs called thrombolytics are often used for this purpose.

Before this kind of treatment can be given, however, caregivers must confirm that the stroke is not hemorrhagic.

Blood thinners can make a hemorrhagic stroke worse and even kill the patient.

Recovering from a Massive Stroke

Recovery from a massive stroke is a long struggle. Complications and resulting impairments become more serious depending on the severity of the stroke. A massive stroke can result in paralysis, loss of muscle control, pain, difficulty with language and speaking, trouble with memory and thinking, and emotional issues.

Rehabilitation services can help minimize complications and may include working with a physical therapist to restore movement, an occupational therapist to learn how to perform daily tasks, a speech therapist to improve speaking ability, and psychologists.

The Long-Term Outlook

The prognosis for a stroke patient depends on the severity of the incident and how quickly medical care is given. The outlook is better for an ischemic stroke. Hemorrhagic strokes have more complications, such as the pressure put on the brain from the ruptured blood vessel.

According to the University of Maryland Medical Center, more than three-quarters of patients survive after the first year, and more than half survive after five years. The odds of survival and recovery become lower with more massive strokes.

Preventing a Stroke

There are risk factors for stroke that can be avoided, and preventive measures that can be taken. Having high blood pressure, drinking too much alcohol, using drugs, and smoking all increase the risk of having a stroke. Being on blood thinners increases the risk of having a hemorrhagic stroke. If you must take blood thinners, speak to your doctor about minimizing your risk of having a stroke.

Risk Factors

New or recurrent strokes affect about 795,000 Americans every year. On average, someone in the United States has a stroke every 40 seconds. While age is the major risk factor, people who have a stroke are likely to have more than one risk factor.

Age: People most at risk for stroke are older adults, particularly those who have high blood pressure, are sedentary, are overweight, smoke, or have diabetes. Older age is also linked with higher rates of post-stroke dementia. Younger people are not immune, however. Many stroke victims are under age 65.

Gender: In most age groups, except older adults, stroke is more common in men than in women. However, stroke kills more women than men. This may be partly due to the fact that women tend to live longer than men, and stroke is more common among older adults. Women account for about 6 in 10 stroke deaths. For younger women, birth control pills and pregnancy can increase the risk of stroke.

Race and Ethnicity: All minority groups, including Native Americans, Hispanics, and African-Americans, face a significantly higher risk for stroke and death from stroke than Caucasians. African-Americans have twice the risk for first-time stroke as Caucasians. The differences in risk among all groups diminish as people age.

The greatest disparity in risk occurs in young adults. Younger African-Americans are two to three times more likely to have a stroke than their Caucasian peers and four times more likely to die from one. They also face a higher risk for death from heart disease. African-Americans have a higher prevalence of obesity, diabetes, and hypertension than other groups. However, studies suggest that socioeconomic factors also affect these differences.

Family History: A family history of stroke or TIA is a strong risk factor for stroke.

Lifestyle Factors: Smoking. People who smoke a pack a day have more than twice the risk for stroke as nonsmokers. Smoking increases both hemorrhagic and ischemic stroke risk. The risk for stroke may remain elevated for as long as 14 years after quitting, so the earlier one quits the better.

Diet: Unhealthy diet (saturated fat, high sodium) can contribute to heart disease, high blood pressure, and obesity, which are all risk factors for stroke.

Physical Inactivity: Lack of regular exercise can increase the risk of obesity, diabetes, and poor circulation, which increase the risk of stroke.

Alcohol and Drug Abuse: Alcohol abuse, including binge drinking, increases the risk of stroke. Drug abuse, particularly with cocaine or methamphetamine, is a major factor of stroke in young adults. Anabolic steroids, used for body-building and sports enhancement, also increase stroke risk.

Heart and Vascular Diseases: Heart disease and stroke are closely tied for many reasons. People who have one heart or vascular condition (such as high blood pressure, high cholesterol, heart disease, diabetes, or peripheral artery disease) are at increased risk for developing other related conditions.

Prior Stroke: A history of a prior stroke or TIA significantly increases the risk for a subsequent stroke. People who have had at least one TIA are 10 times more likely to have a stroke than those who have not had a TIA.

Prior Heart Attack: People who have had a heart attack are at increased risk of stroke.

High Blood Pressure: High blood pressure (hypertension) contributes to about 70% of all strokes. People with hypertension have up to 10 times the normal risk of stroke, depending on the severity of the blood pressure and the presence of other risk factors. Hypertension is also an important cause of so-called silent cerebral infarcts ("mini-strokes" caused by blockages in the blood vessels in the brain), which may predict major stroke. Controlling blood pressure is extremely important for stroke prevention.

Unhealthy Cholesterol Levels: A high total cholesterol level increases the risk of developing atherosclerosis ("hardening of the arteries") and heart disease. In atherosclerosis, fatty deposits (plaques) of cholesterol build up in the arteries of the heart.

Heart Disease: Coronary artery disease (heart disease), which is the end result of atherosclerosis, increases stroke risk. Anti-clotting medications, which are used in heart disease treatment to break up blood clots, can increase the risk of hemorrhagic stroke.

Atrial Fibrillation: A major risk factor for stroke, is a heart rhythm disorder in which the atria (the upper chambers in the heart) beat very rapidly and irregularly. The blood stagnates instead of being pumped out promptly, increasing the risk for formation of blood clots that break loose and travel toward the brain. Between 2 - 4% of patients with atrial fibrillation without any history of TIA or stroke will have an ischemic stroke over the course of a year. The risk is generally highest for those older than age 75, with heart failure or enlarged heart, coronary artery disease, history of clots, diabetes, or heart valve abnormalities.

Structural Heart Problems: Dilated cardiomyopathy (enlarged heart), heart valve disorders, and congenital heart defects, such as patent foramen ovalae (opening in chambers of heart) and atrial septal aneurysm (bulging of heart chamber), are risk factors for stroke.

Carotid Artery Disease and Peripheral Artery Disease: is a serious risk factor for stroke. Atherosclerosis can cause fatty build-up in the carotid arteries of the neck, which can lead to blood clots that block blood flow and oxygen to the brain. People with peripheral artery disease, which occurs when atherosclerosis narrows blood vessels in the legs and arms, are at increased risk of carotid artery disease and subsequently stroke.

Hypertension: is a disorder characterized by chronically high blood pressure. It must be monitored, treated, and controlled by medication, lifestyle changes, or a combination of both.

Diabetes: Heart disease and stroke are the leading causes of death in people with diabetes. Diabetes is second only to high blood pressure as the main risk factor for stroke. The risk is highest for adults newly diagnosed with type 2 diabetes and patients with diabetes who are younger than age 55. African-Americans with diabetes are at even higher risk for stroke at a younger age. Diabetes is a particularly strong risk factor for ischemic stroke, perhaps because of accompanying risk factors such as obesity and high blood pressure. Diabetes does not appear to increase the risk for hemorrhagic stroke.

Obesity and Metabolic Syndrome: Obesity may increase the risk for both ischemic and hemorrhagic stroke independently of other risk factors that often co-exist with excess weight, including diabetes, high blood pressure, and unhealthy cholesterol level. Weight that is centered around the abdomen (the so-called apple shape) has a particularly high association with stroke, as it does for heart disease, in comparison to weight distributed around hips (pear-shape).

Obesity is particularly hazardous when it is one of the components of metabolic syndrome. This syndrome is diagnosed when three of the following conditions are present: abdominal obesity, low HDL cholesterol, high triglyceride levels, high blood pressure, and insulin resistance. Because metabolic syndrome is a pre-diabetic condition that is significantly associated with heart disease, people with this syndrome are at increased risk for stroke even before diabetes develops.

Other Risk Factors: Migraine. Studies suggest that migraine or severe headache may be a risk factor for stroke in both men and women, especially before age 50. Overall, 2 - 3% of ischemic strokes occur in people with a history of migraine. However, in patients under age 45, about 15% of all strokes (and 30 - 60% of strokes in young women) are associated with a history of migraines, particularly migraine with aura. For young women with migraines, other risk factors (such as high blood pressure, smoking, and use of estrogen-containing oral contraceptives) may increase stroke risk.

Sickle Cell Disease: People with sickle cell disease are at increased risk for stroke at a young age.

Pregnancy: carries a very small risk for stroke, mostly in women with pregnancy-related high blood pressure. The risk appears to be higher in the postpartum (post-delivery) period, perhaps because of the sudden change in circulation and hormone levels.

Depression: Some research suggests that depression may increase the risk for stroke.

NSAIDs: Nonsteroidal anti-inflammatory drugs (NSAIDs) such as ibuprofen (Advil, Motrin, generic) and diclofenac (Cataflam, Voltaren, generic) may increase the risk of stroke, especially for patients who have other stroke risk factors.

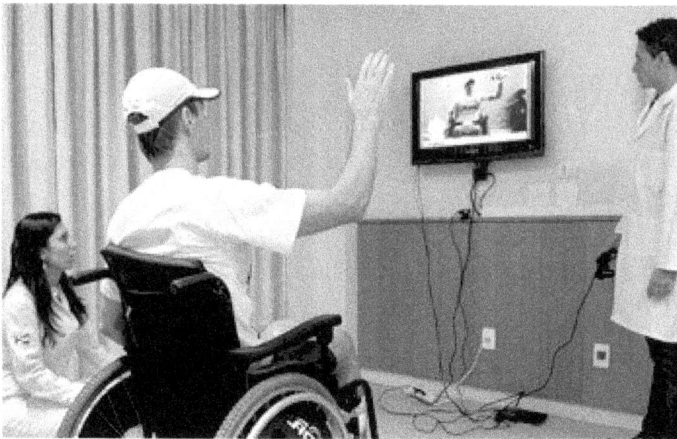

Stroke victim in therapy session.

Prognosis

Stroke is the fourth leading cause of death in the United States. Mortality rates are declining, however. Over 75% of patients survive a first stroke during the first year, and over half survive beyond 5 years.

Severity of an Ischemic Versus Hemorrhagic Stroke

People who suffer ischemic strokes have a much better chance for survival than those who have hemorrhagic strokes. Among the ischemic stroke categories, the greatest dangers are posed by embolic strokes, followed by thrombotic and lacunar strokes.

Hemorrhagic stroke not only destroys brain cells but also poses other complications, including increased pressure on the brain or spasms in the blood vessels, both of which can be very dangerous. Studies suggest, however, that survivors of hemorrhagic stroke have a greater chance for recovering function than those who survive ischemic stroke.

Long-Term Complications and Disabilities

Many patients are left with physical weakness and often have accompanying pain and spasticity (muscle stiffness or spasms). Depending on the severity of the symptoms and how much of the body is involved, these impairments can affect the ability to walk, to rise from a chair, to feed oneself, to write or use a computer, to drive, and many other activities.

Factors that Affect Quality of Life in Survivors

Many stroke survivors recover functional independence after a stroke, but 25% are left with a minor disability and 40% experience moderate-to-severe disabilities. The National Institutes of Health (NIH)'s stroke scale helps predict the severity and outcome of a stroke by scoring 11 factors (levels of consciousness, gaze, visual fields, facial movement, motor functions in the arm and leg, coordination, sensory loss, problems with language, inability to articulate, and attention).

Patients with ischemic strokes who score less than 10 have a favorable outlook after a year, while only 4 - 16% of patients do well if their score is more than 20.

Factors Affecting Recurrence

The risk for recurring stroke is highest within the first few weeks and months of the previous stroke. But about 25% of people who have a first stroke will go on to have another stroke within 5 years. Risk factors for recurrence include:

- Older age
- Evidence of blocked arteries (a history of coronary artery disease, carotid artery disease, peripheral artery disease, ischemic stroke, or TIA)
- Hemorrhagic or embolic stroke
- Diabetes
- Alcoholism
- Valvular heart disease
- Atrial fibrillation

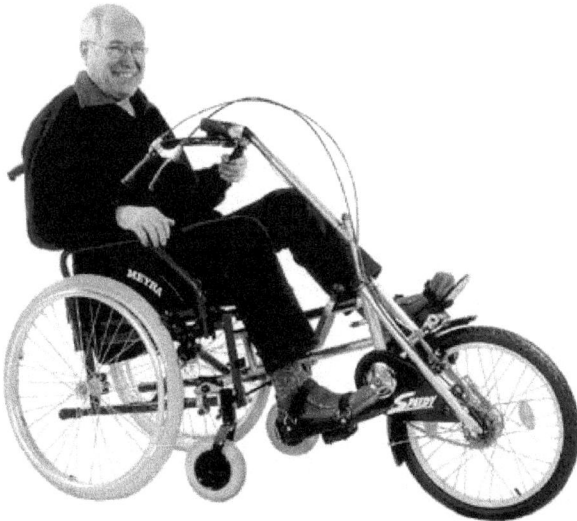

Foot pedals on wheelchair for mobility and exercise.

Managing Stroke Complications

In the days following stroke, patients are at risk for complications. The below steps are important.

- **Maintain Adequate Delivery of Oxygen:** It is very important to maintain oxygen levels. In some cases, airway ventilation may be required. Supplemental oxygen may also be necessary for patients when tests suggest low blood levels of oxygen. *[Steve Hatch had slept for several years with oxygen at night for COPD/emphysema yet when he entered the care center 16 days after being released from Mercy Medical Center in Sioux City, Iowa after being stabilized from the stroke, Blackhawk Life Care Center in Lake View, Iowa didn't have an oxygen concentrator for him. I was alarmed during one of my first visits at the care center when I found him was laying in bed gasping for air. I reported it to the nurse's station and they said they only had orders to put it on at night when he was sleeping but she said she would turn it on. I felt so sorry for the alarmed look he had on his face and eyes looking at me as he was gasping for air. MJW]*

- **Manage Fever:** Fever should be monitored and aggressively treated with medication and, if needed, a cooling blanket since its presence predicts a poorer outlook.

- **Evaluate Swallowing:** Patients should have their swallowing function evaluated before they are given any food, fluid, or medication by mouth. If patients cannot adequately swallow they are at risk of choking. Patients who cannot swallow on their own may require nutrition and fluids delivered intravenously or through a tube placed in the nose or the stomach.

- **Maintain Electrolytes:** Maintaining a healthy electrolyte balance (the ratio of sodium, calcium, and potassium in the body's fluids) is critical.

- **Control Blood Pressure:** Managing blood pressure is essential but complicated. Blood pressure often declines spontaneously in the first 24 hours after stroke. Patients whose blood pressure remains elevated should be treated carefully with antihypertensive medications.
- **Monitor Increased Brain Pressure:** Hospital staff should watch closely for evidence of increased pressure on the brain (cerebral edema), which is a frequent complication of hemorrhagic strokes. It can also occur a few days after ischemic strokes. Early symptoms of increased brain pressure are drowsiness, confusion, lethargy, weakness, and headache. Medications such as mannitol may be given during a stroke to reduce pressure or the risk for it.
- **Elevated the Heat:** Keeping the top of the body higher than the lower part, such as by elevating the head of the bed, can reduce pressure in the brain and is standard practice for patients with ischemic stroke. However, this practice also lowers blood pressure in general, which may be dangerous for patients with massive stroke.
- **Monitor the Heart:** Patients must be monitored using electrocardiographic tracings to check for atrial fibrillation and other heart rhythm problems. Patients are at high risk for heart attack following stroke.
- **Control Blood Sugar (Glucose) Levels**: Elevated blood sugar (glucose) levels can occur with severe stroke and may be a marker of serious trouble. Patients with high blood glucose levels may require insulin therapy.
- **Monitor Blood Coagulation:** Regular tests for blood coagulation are important to make sure that the blood is not so "thick" that it will clot nor so "thin" that it causes bleeding.
- **Check for Deep Venous Thrombosis:** Deep venous thrombosis is a blood clot in the veins of the lower leg or thigh. It can be a serious post-stroke complication because there is a risk of the clot breaking off and

traveling to the brain or heart. Deep venous thrombosis can also cause pulmonary embolism if the blood clot travels to the lungs. If necessary, an anticoagulant drug such as heparin may be given, but this increases the risk of hemorrhage. Patients who have had a stroke are also at risk for pulmonary embolisms

• **Prevent Infection:** Patients who have had a stroke are at increased risk for pneumonia, urinary tract infections, and other widespread infections.

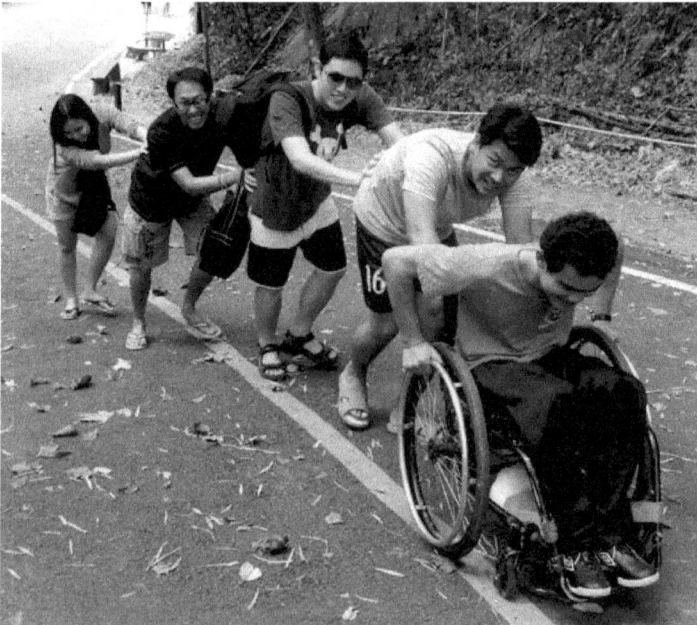

↳Friends having fun, look at those smiles.

Prevention and Rehabilitation Programs

Patients who have had a first stroke or TIA are at high risk of having another stroke. Secondary prevention measures are essential to reduce this risk.

Limit Alcohol Consumption. Heavy alcohol use and binge drinking increase the risk of both ischemic and hemorrhagic stroke. If you drink, limit alcohol to no more than one drink a day for women or two drinks a day for men.

Rehabilitation Programs

Because stroke affects different parts of the brain, specific approaches to managing rehabilitation vary widely among individual patients:

Exercise program: Guidelines from the Veteran's Administration recommend that patients get back on their feet as soon as possible to prevent deep vein thrombosis. Patients should try to walk at least 50 feet a day. Assisted devices or bracing are sometimes used to help support the legs. Treadmill exercises can be very helpful for patients with mild-to-moderate dysfunction. Exercise should be tailored to the stroke survivor's physical condition and can include aerobic, strength, flexibility, and neuromuscular (coordination and balance) activities.

Retraining muscles: Stretching and range-of-motion exercises are used to help treat spastic muscles. They can also help patients regain function in a paralyzed arm. Multiple techniques have been developed and studied.

Speech therapy and sign language: Intense speech therapy after a stroke is important for recovery. Some doctors recommend 9 hours a week of therapy for 3 months. Language skills improve the most when family and **friends** help reinforce the speech therapy lessons. *[Steve Hatch received no speech therapy other than being analyzed for not being able to speak. MJW]*

Swallowing training: Training patients **and their caregivers** regarding swallowing techniques, as well as safe and not-safe foods and liquids, is essential for preventing aspiration (accidental sucking in of food or fluids into the airway). *[I could have helped Steve Hatch with swallowing exercises but I was completely isolated from any care or discussion on his therapy. MJW]*

Attention training: Problems with attention are very common after strokes. Direct retraining teaches patients to perform specific tasks using repetitive drills in response to certain stimuli. (For example, they are told to press a buzzer each time they hear a specific number.) A variant of this approach trains patients to relearn real-life skills, such as driving, carrying on a conversation, or other daily tasks.

Occupational training: Occupational therapy is important and improves daily living activities and social participation.

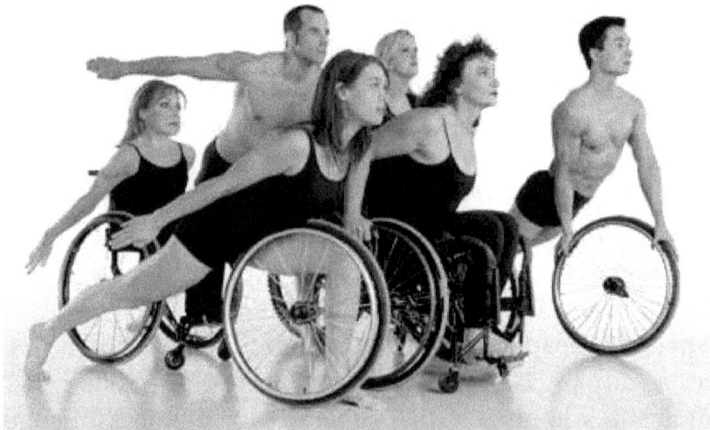

Dance troupe incorporates two paralyzed dancers.

Therapy for Swallowing

Exercises to help regain swallowing after stroke. Dysphagia is an impairment in the ability to swallow due to strokes and other injuries to the central and peripheral nervous systems. Dysphagia can be benign and rapidly curable, but it can also be rapidly progressive and even deadly.

Swallowing is a complicated neurological reflex that involves a well orchestrated sequence of three major phases. These begin in the mouth with the coordinated action of muscles involved with chewing and the formation of a food bolus, a small and soft mass of food. This is followed by the transfer of this food bolus towards the pharynx, where it triggers an automatic sequence of movements of several small muscles that then work together to channel the food into the esophagus, the "food pipe" which finally brings food to the stomach. All this must occur while preventing food or liquid particles from entering the lungs.

Swallowing And The Brain

The brain is a complex organ in which different areas are designated for the control of different functions -- and swallowing is no exception. In fact, there are multiple brain areas dedicated to the control of swallowing. Damage to one or more of these areas, as can happen with stroke, can lead to dysphagia.

When Is a Feeding Tube Really Necessary?

Sometimes dysphagia is so severe that it requires the temporary, or even permanent, placement of a feeding tube. Although at first the decision to agree to have a feeding tube placed by your doctor might seem straight forward, it rarely is. In fact, deciding whether or not you should agree to the placement of a feeding tube (for you or someone else) can be an extremely difficult task. Talk with your doctor, or your loved one's physician (if you're a caretaker), about the possibility of this being a necessity.

Shaker Exercise

Lie flat on your back and raise your head as though you were trying to fixate your gaze on your toes. While you do this, make sure not to raise your shoulders. This simple exercise improves swallowing ability if it is performed three to six times per day for at least six weeks. If you get good at it, increase the duration of each head lift and the number of repetitions.

Hyoid Lift Maneuver

This is a rather simple exercise, although it may sound more like a task performed in one of those reality TV shows. Place a few small pieces of paper (about 1 inch in diameter) over a blanket or a towel.

Then place a straw in your mouth and suck one of the pieces of paper to its tip. Keep sucking on the straw to keep the paper attached, bring it over a cup or a similar container and stop sucking. This will release the paper into the container. Your goal is to place about 5 to 10 pieces of paper into the container.

Mendelsohn Maneuver

This simple exercise is very effective at improving the swallowing reflex. It involves swallowing your own saliva. Normally, as the saliva enters the area just behind your mouth during swallowing, your "Adam's apple" (the hard area about halfway down the front of your neck) moves up and then back down. To do this exercise, keep the Adam's apple elevated for about 2 to 5 seconds each time.

You can help it stay there with your fingers at first, in order to better understand the movement you are about to do. But the exercise will only help you once you can make it stay up without assistance. Repeat this exercise several times per day.

Effortful Swallow

The purpose of this exercise is to improve the contact among the different muscles used during the act of swallowing. In essence, the exercise consists of swallowing. But as you do it, you must try to squeeze all of the muscles of swallowing as hard as you can. You do not need to swallow food during the exercise. Just a dry swallow will do. Perform this exercise 5 to 10 times, 3 times per day.

Supraglottic Swallow

You should try this exercise without food first. As you get good at it, you can try it with actual food in your mouth. This exercise consists of 3 simple steps. First, take a deep breath. Hold it as you swallow, then cough to clear any residues of saliva or food which might have gone down past your vocal cords.

Super Supraglottic Swallow Maneuver

This exercise is just like the supraglottic maneuver described above, but with an extra twist. After you take that deep breath, bear down while swallowing. The pressure generated helps with swallowing and increases the strength of your swallowing muscles.

Your ability to swallow can be weakened after a stroke. This problem is called dysphagia. While it may sound like a bothersome problem, swallowing trouble is actually more dangerous than it is annoying. Most stroke survivors who have problems with swallowing impairment do not notice that it is difficult to swallow food and drinks, but instead experience problems such as choking and coughing up food.

Swallowing problems cause the risk of a serious side effect, which is aspiration.

What is Aspiration?

Aspiration means that food, drinks or even saliva can go down the wrong pipe towards the lungs instead of towards the stomach, potentially causing trouble breathing or a lung infection called pneumonia.

Aspiration occurs when the misrouted liquid or bits of food block air from getting into the lungs. This can cause a bout of coughing, which is a reflex that occurs to try to dislodge the droplets of liquid or food particles from irritating the throat and obstructing air. When aspiration is severe, excessive material in the lungs may irritate the lungs and cause pneumonia, which is a type of lung infection.

How Does Aspiration Occur?

Your mouth directs food to the esophagus, which leads to the stomach. Your nose and mouth also direct air to the lungs. After food or air enters the mouth, a small passageway (the pharynx) takes in air and food, and then divides to send food down a food pipe (the esophagus) to the stomach or air down a windpipe (the larynx) to the lungs.

Under normal circumstances, a small structure called the epiglottis closes off the windpipe when we swallow to prevent food from going down the wrong pipe.

Aspiration occurs when food, liquids or even saliva enter the windpipe instead of the food pipe. This can happen during swallowing, or the material may even come back up after going down the correct tube, and enter into the wrong tube.

Why Does a Stroke Cause Aspiration?

Swallowing, which we often take for granted, requires perfect coordination of a number of different muscles controlled by the brain. A stroke affects the muscles involved in swallowing, often preventing proper chewing and swallowing so that food enters the wrong tube.

Sometimes, after a stroke, food that has begun to go down the correct tube may return back up and enter the wrong tube.

A stroke may even cause the swallowing muscles to weaken in such a way that saliva may leak down into the wrong pipe- even if you aren't actively eating. Normally, our bodies produce saliva, and we reflexively swallow to decrease the buildup in our mouths.

One recent clinical research study used a video recording to evaluate stroke patients and demonstrated that the esophagus remains open for a longer period of time with swallowing, possibly allowing material an excessive opportunity to go down the wrong pipe.

Another research study found that stroke survivors who have larger strokes and strokes that affect the right side of the brain (the non-dominant side) experience more serious swallowing problems.

What Can You Do?

Managing swallowing problems on your own is not recommended, as swallowing is a complex skill. A speech and swallow evaluation is necessary after a stroke, even if you have not noticed obvious problems with swallowing. Your speech and swallow therapist will recommend foods and liquids of a safe consistency and will also provide you with exercises and a plan to help you advance to other foods.

Some safety recommendations include sitting up at a 90 degree angle during and after meals, pacing yourself as you eat and drink, cutting the food into small pieces and avoiding other activities such as talking, while eating. Some people with severe swallowing problems may sleep in a non-flat position to avoid aspiration.

Swallowing problems are not usually the most obvious handicap after a stroke. But, like bladder problems that may occur after a stroke, swallowing difficulties can interfere with your quality of life and can even cause serious health consequences. Taking good care of yourself after a stroke includes getting attention for the subtle effects of your stroke.

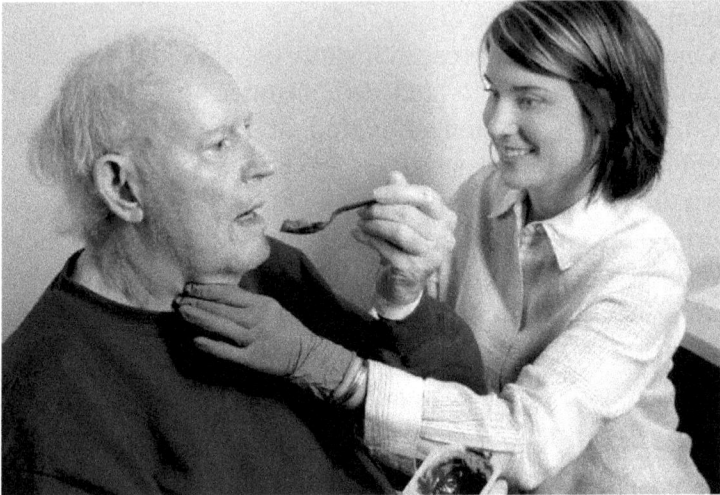

Therapist checking for swallowing problems.

Inventions and Aids for Stroke Victims

Computer Apps for Stroke Survivors

If the person is able to hold an iPad, there are apps online that can be installed to help the person communicate by touching simple icons on the screen.

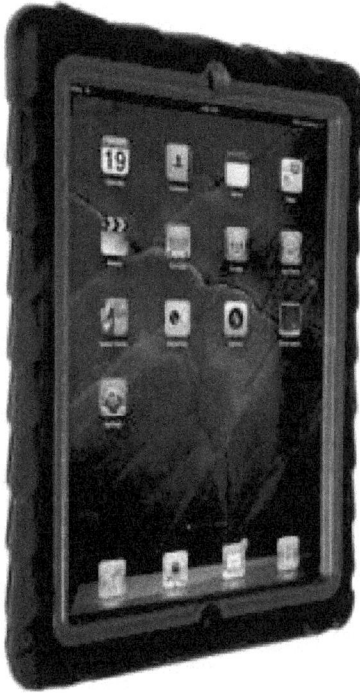

If they are unable to hold the device and touch the screen, there are pads to hold tablets.

A ThaiPad from Levenger is a padded pyramid-shaped pillow to support books, tablets, and ebook readers. It would be soft enough to be put on lap or on the person's chest as they lay in bed.

A fun way to work on fine motor control and reasoning skills would be a "Chalk Board"-- a simple drawing program. There are also games like Hangman or Tic-tac-toe or

Montessori Crosswords -- a spelling game for children. These games would prove more interesting than actually pushing letter tiles around on a tabletop as the patient works on their fine motor control without being bored.

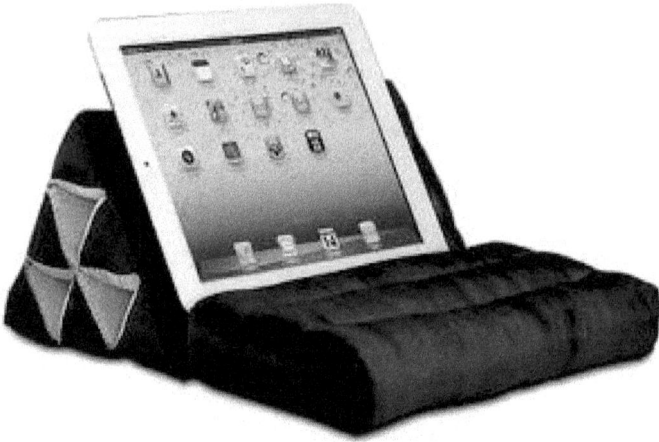

The videos are easy to see in the small window and remain clear and to easy to use on various screens.

A Wii Fit Board helps senior citizens maintain and improve their physical abilities. It should also work as well for stroke patients to improve their strength and balance as the iPad helps with fine motor control and speech.

Touch Voice produces three medical grade speaking software apps which run on various computer Android tablets, iPads, some smart phones, most laptops and desktops allowing the speech impaired to speak by touching or clicking on buttons.

Touch Voice apps have been designed to address medical conditions such as Stroke, ALS, Traumatic Brain Injury, Brain Tumor, Cerebral Palsy, Multiple Sclerosis, Ataxia, Dysarthria, Laryngeal Cancer and potentially others not listed here.

People who can't speak are frustrated trying to communicate with their caregivers, friends, family and loved ones. Just as others can be frustrated in trying to communicate with them. For some their speech may be just too weak or inarticulate to understand. By using Touch Voice Apps they can quickly and easily voice their needs and feelings, thereby better communicating in general. Ultimately this can reduce their stress levels, lead to better care and aid in their recovery.

It is important to understand the appropriateness of Touch Voice AAC software apps, and that their use may be different in every situation, medical condition, and specific individual. We recommend larger tablets with large touch surfaces over phones and computer devices. This is due to an associative nature of speech impairment in which in some cases, hands and fingers may be too shaky or weak to touch the smaller buttons which speak words.

In other cases, cognitive damage to word recognition makes it difficult to communicate, so we have included images with words to assist those individuals. A NEW Touch Voice Gold works on most devices (iPads 2 and above, Android devices, Microsoft and Apple computers.)

The healthcare industry and the broader field of technology have complimented each other for many years, so it's no surprise that thanks to recent advancements in technology, here has been an emergence of 3D technology in the field of rehabilitation. Simple put, this is great news – with 3D rehab technology, the world will be a much better place for those of us on the mend. Like many other forms of scientific advancements, a number of options are available for those looking to use 3D rehab technology. The most innovative and beneficial forms of 3D rehab technology are treadmills, simulators and also a few that utilize the video game console known as the Nintendo Wii. Here's what you should know about each!

Anti-Gravity Treadmill

The first rehab technology source that one can use is the anti-gravity treadmill. This is simply a kind of treadmill that uses air pressure to help record a more precise measurement of body weight. As a result ,the person in rehab will have the ability to measure anywhere between 20 to 100% of body weight used to walk and run. People who are recovering from spinal cord injuries, surgery or athletic strain will benefit most from this particular technology.

Weight-Supported Treadmill

You should also know about the body-weight supported treadmills. These allow people to use proper posture while having their body weight supported. As a result, users will have a way to walk and run faster. The treadmill provides ease of movement and rhythmic motions to help a person improve and enhance their ability to move on a regular basis. Like the anti-gravity treadmills, this will benefit people who are training for athletic events, as well as recovering from trauma or surgery.

Nintendo Wii Console

Perhaps the most interesting of these new tools is the Nintendo Wii. This video game console offers a number of games that people can play that require physical movement. This can be arguably the most fun rehab technology product on the market, due to the variety of games that you can play. These games focus on everything from aerobics to agility. This is arguably the most innovative and practical 3D rehab technology device on the market.

Fes-Bike

The FES bike is an exercise bike that operates much better than most. It can provide a 3D screen that will help monitor progress as well as give users a very clear template of their workouts. This bike helps stimulate up to six muscle groups of the legs and therefore allows people to develop endurance and stamina for the lower body. People who are recovering from knee surgery or calf injuries, and also those who run and cycle will benefit most from this form of technology

Thanks to the development of 3D rehab technology, many people will have practical and efficient options to take advantage of when looking to enhance their strength and stamina. It's also ideal for those looking to recover from a number of injuries due to its state of the art design, efficiency and also versatility. Anyone looking to take advantage of technology that will help them recover from injuries as well as enhance their physical performance will benefit by jumping on this train ASAP!

Wii Fit hula game

Recovering stroke patient gets into the rhythm of a
Wii Fit hula game with the help of the physical therapist.

Patient reacting to Wii Fi monitor for exercise and
rehabilitation.

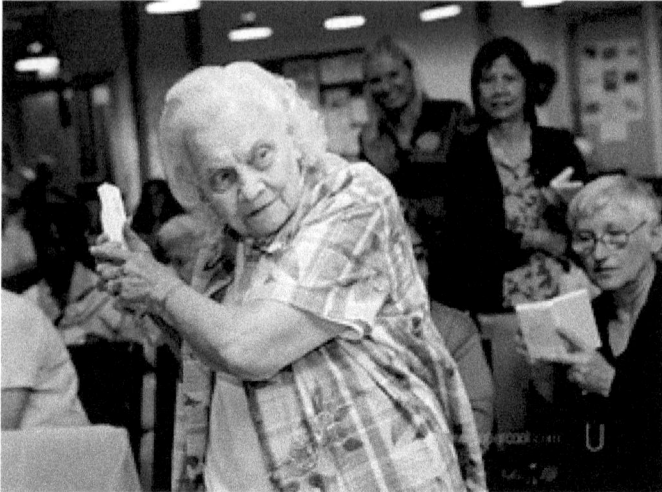

Who can use the Wii?

Just about anyone can use the Wii from young children to senior citizens. There are some physical requirements necessary, but even some of them, such as the ability to grasp a controller can be accommodated for. A patient will need to have some control of upper extremity movement to use the games requiring the Wii remote. In order to use the Wii Fit Balance Board the patient will need some lower extremity strength (enough to stand) if they are going to stand on the board, or some core strength if they are going to sit on the board.

Why does Wiihab work?

Wiihab creates an environment for the patient in which they can take their mind off the burden of the rehabilitation process while they are participating in it. The patient is motivated by either accomplishing goals in the games they participate in or by competing with another patient in rehab. The game draws the patient in and within time they forget they are exercising. A therapist that is careful choosing which games to play can plan a successful workout.

Setup

The equipment is easy to set up and once all of the cords are plugged in the patient or therapist can control the game from the Wii remote. The only time someone would need to help the patients with the console is if a game disk needed to be changed out. By choosing a game like Wii Sports or Wii fit there are multiple games on one disk to keep the patients challenged.

Exercise programs

There are a variety of games for the Wii that are specifically designed for exercise. Wii sports includes tennis, bowling, boxing, golf, and baseball. Some of the sports are more physically challenging than others just as they are in real life. Bowling requires more coordination than physical exertion. While boxing requires a lot of movement but does not rely on a high degree of accuracy. Someone that is interested in using a Wii for rehab should play the games and decide which games would work best for the particular patient and muscle groups they are trying to strengthen.

Wiihab Different Parts of the Body

The Arms

Most games for the Wii are great for exercising the arms. Games that are sports related tend to focus on using real life movements required in those sports to make the characters in the game move. Boxing and tennis games require a lot of quick movements. Patients that need upper extremity strengthening can start out playing the game with just a controller and then move up to having weights added to their arms to provide more resistance.

Repetitive motion games such as running require the subject to shake the Wii remote. The shaking motion strengthens the endurance of the patient. It is important that the physical therapist or person in charge of the rehabilitation watches the amount of repetition that various joints receive. There have been tendinitis injuries caused by children playing the Wii for to many hours at a time.

Mini games seen in games like Mario Party offer a good balance of repetitive motion activities. While the patient is navigating the game board they are essentially resting their arms, but during a mini game they are experiencing a little session of intense exercise.

The Legs

The legs can be exercised in a couple of ways. First they can be exercised by simulating movements such as running or jumping as required by a game. An example of this would be Jillian Michael's Fitness Ultimatum game for the Wii. In this game the patient is asked to jog from one exercise station to the next. The Wii does not actually know if the patient is jogging. It detects movement through the Wii remote and attached Nunchuk. So the patient can stand and jog or pretend to jog by just moving their arms.

The legs can also be exercised through the use of the Wii Fit balance board. The Wii Fit balance board can detect changes in force which translate into center of pressure movements. Movements in the center or pressure control the character on the screen. In Wii fit, the game that comes with the balance board, there are a variety of games that contribute to leg strengthening such as step aerobics, balance games, yoga, and strength training exercises.

The Core

The core can be strengthened by a lot of the balance games and yoga positions in Wii Fit. The game starts outeasy and even analyzes a patients initial balance. As the patient gets better the games become harder or longer thus requiring an increased response from the patient.

The Mind

The games are also mentally stimulating. They sometimes require logic and problem solving skills. There are a variety of mini games included in Mario Party and Carnival Games for the Wii which require the patient to memorize patterns and then repeat the pattern back. These same games can also help with patient's dexterity and coordination by requiring the patient to conduct fine movements of objects on the screen using the Wii remote. One such mini game in Carnival games requires the subject to move a ring through a wire maze without touching the ring to the wire. If they do then the Wii remote vibrates and they have to start over again.

Using the Wii to Chart Progress

Inherently built into the Wii is the ability to save game data for multiple players, depending on the game. The nice thing about saving progress and recording high scores is the ability to compare scores from the same patient over a particular time period. A patient that has never used a Wii will first have to get comfortable with the controller and how it responds to their movements. After this initial learning curve is overcome the patients true coordination and strength progress can be assessed. As a patient improves harder levels can be tried or new games can be added to the workout.

Wii Fit Plus comes with a built in personal training schedule which allows the player to choose a custom workout schedule that they can do everyday. The software tracks their score and times to complete certain activities and gives the patient workout activities based on their current abilities. If a patient is able to sit or stand on the balance board then software is also able to calculate changes in their body weight and graph it on the screen. A patient that may need to lose weight can input a weight loss goal and the Wii Fit software can track their progress.

One downside is that while progress can be tracked not all games have this feature. Another problem is that currently if the data needs to be stored in the patients chart it needs to be hand written, unlike a computer there is not a way to send the data to a printer.

The Use of Wiihab With Different Disabilities

Stroke: In a case study published in the International Journal of Rehabilitation Research, investigators found that Wii fit was beneficial for an 86 year old poststroke patient. It improved her balance and improved her gait confidence. They used the Timed Up and Go (TUG) outcome measure and found a 10 second time improvement after the patient exercised using four of the balance games in Wii fit during four training sessions.

Cerebral Palsy: Researchers used three outcome measures to determine if Wiihab was helpful in rehabilitation. The three outcome measures used were:

1) Visual-perceptual processing, using a motor-free perceptual test (Test of Visual Perceptual Skills, third edition)
2) Postural control, using weight distribution and sway measures
3) Functional mobility, using gait distance.

All three outcomes showed improvements after training.

Traumatic Brain Injury (TBI)

Acquired brain injury therapists at UPMC Mercy Hospital found that 1 hour Wiihab sessions with Traumatic Brain Injury patients helped in three ways:

1) Improved hand eye coordination.
2) Improved social participation.
3) Reduced feelings of helplessness.

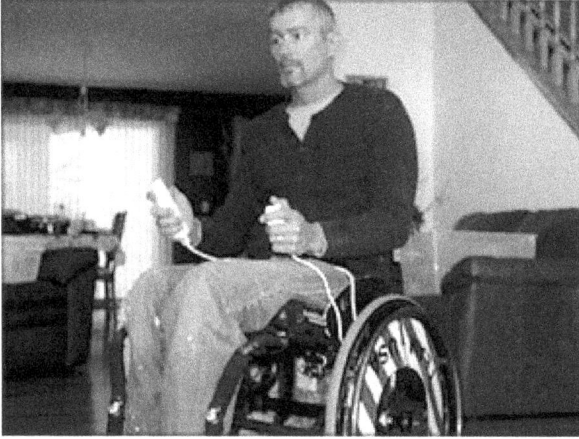

They did not report on outcome measures used, but expressed their clinical observation.

Amputees

Ossur conducted a study using Wii fit to determine which exercises would be helpful or difficult for a transtibial or transfemoral amputee to participate in. A manual specific to lower extremity amputees was designed (not included here).

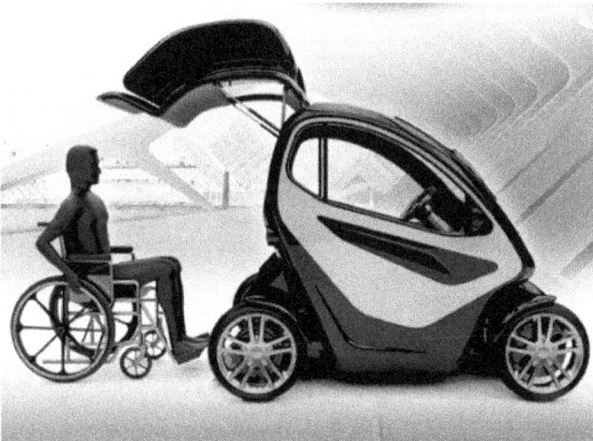

Roll-in motor-vehicle. One person operation and street legal in most smaller towns.

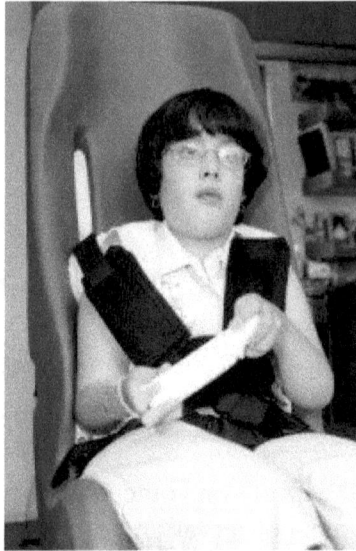

A little over a year ago doctors in Canada thought of using the Nintendo Wii, which had been used as entertainment for young spinal cord injury recovering patients, and as therapy for patients after strokes. What they began to realize is that this system, the Nintendo Wii, could be just what is needed to help with rehabilitation because of its ease of use and friendly interface. Some of the things it will help them with is the balance, eye coordination, with memory, problem solving, etc.

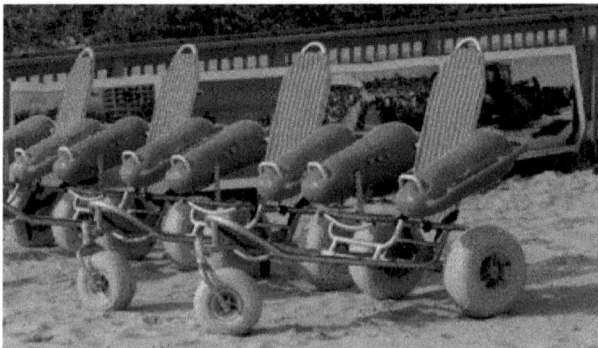

Beach and water chairs available at many handicap-accessible beaches.

Physical Rehab Equipment for strengthening legs

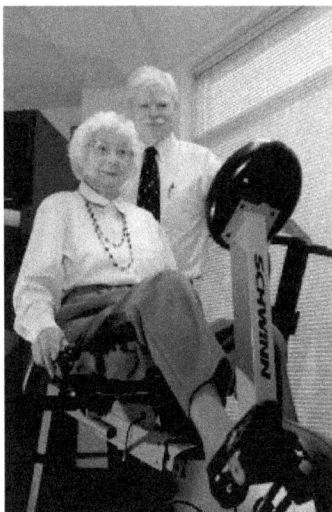

Woman exercising her legs. The active leg helps stimulate
the paralyzed leg/foot to improve nerves and blood flow.

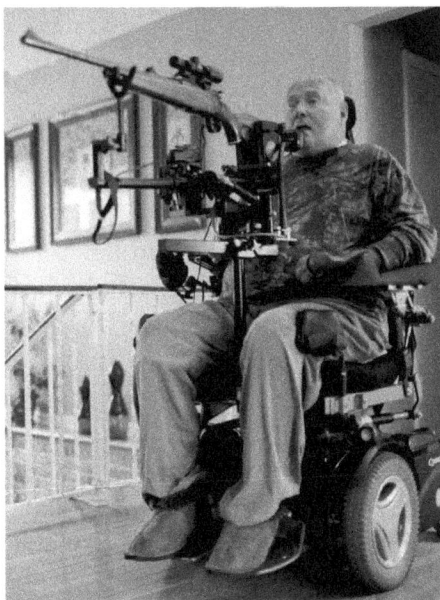

Paralyzed man ready for hunting in his electric wheelchair.

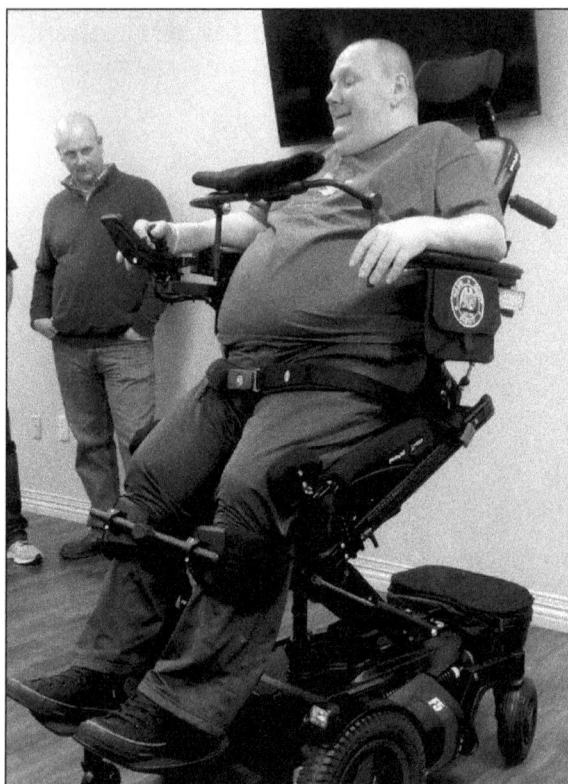

Completely paralyzed man in "standup" electric wheelchair. Finger controls, seatbelt, headrest front and back. Do you see this man's smile? There is life after stroke.

When I took my mother to the hospital when she was being treated for cancer, all they offered her to sit in while getting checked in to the outpatient area to have a JPEG (stomach feeding tube) installed was a standard wheel chair. She was too weak to hold her head up so I had to stand behind her in the waiting room and let her rest her head in my cupped hands as I stood behind the wheelchair. Head rests should be optional equipment for all wheelchairs – either removable or adjustable.

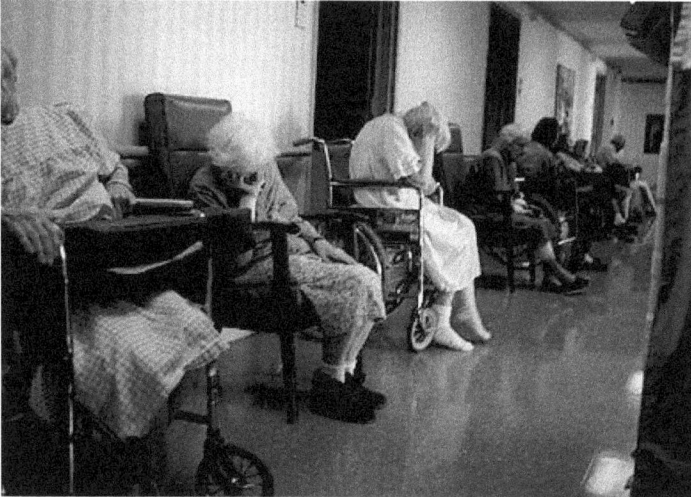

This is what real nursing homes look like. Do those chairs look comfortable for long periods of time? Some of the ladies are tied in so they don't fall out of their chairs. A headrest and/or slightly reclining seats would greatly improve their comfort.

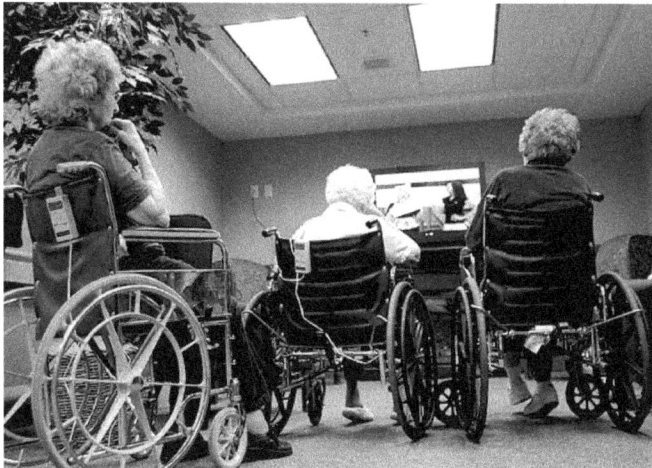

These women appear to be fairly mobile and able to wheel themselves around to watch TV. But how hard would it be to make wheelchairs with extended back so they could lay their heads back if they wanted. I get a neck ache just looking at how low the back of the wheelchairs are where they are cutting into their backs. Think how difficult it would be for a large man completely paralyzed on one side try to sit upright in a one-size-fits-all wheelchair that would cut into his back only lower with no place for him to rest his head supported by weakened/paralyzed neck muscles.

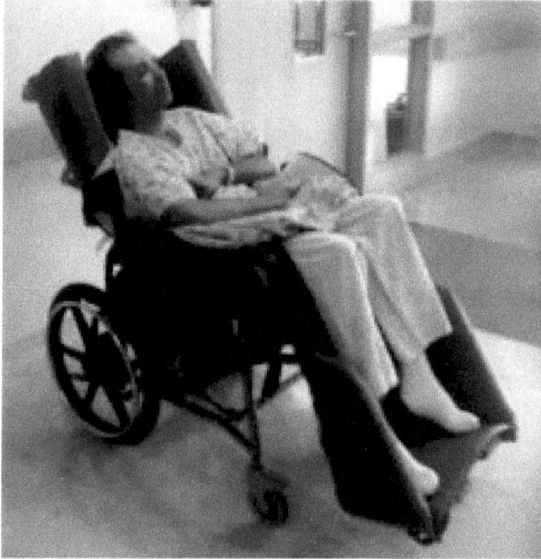

Shown above is a wheelchair for paralyzed people. The sides will keep the body centered along with a place to rest their head. Also note that the toes are protected via a platform from being bashed against a doorway, furniture, or being pushing into other obstructions. The more pictures I see of modern wheelchairs designed for handicapped people, the more I believe the medical profession is still operating in the ice age for the majority of their patients.

I find it hard to believe that 99% of hospitals and nursing homes do not offer slightly-reclining wheelchairs with a headrest. A person who is paralyzed on one side from a stroke also has affected or weakened nerves and muscles in their neck. It is cruel and inhuman treatment to expect them to sit for long hours without an option for them to rest their head against a head rest if they need to.

If you think this is an isolated incidence, go to a nursing home and see how many old people are sitting in the hallways in wheelchairs with their heads slumped clear down on their chest. I don't see how they can even breathe much less be comfortable or able to straighten their neck after a period of time sitting like that.

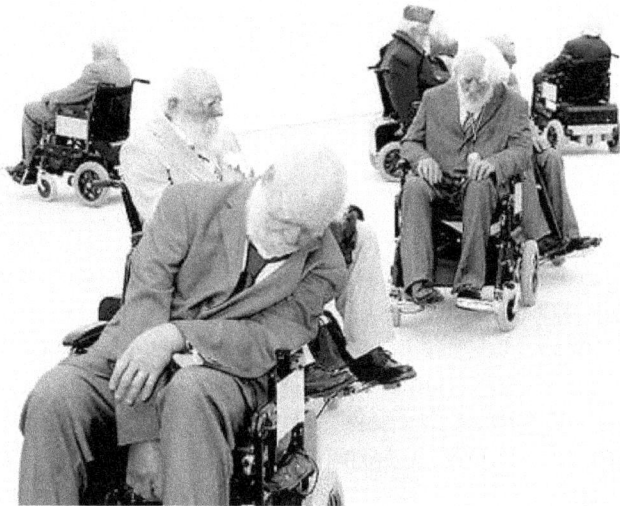

Vision of old men slumped in wheel chairs. This is actually a staged work of art. But the motivation for this display is the reality of what people look like who are left sitting in traditional wheel chairs without head rests and no adjustment to slightly recline. A paralyzed person will eventually slide down and to the weakened side without the strength or ability to straighten upright.

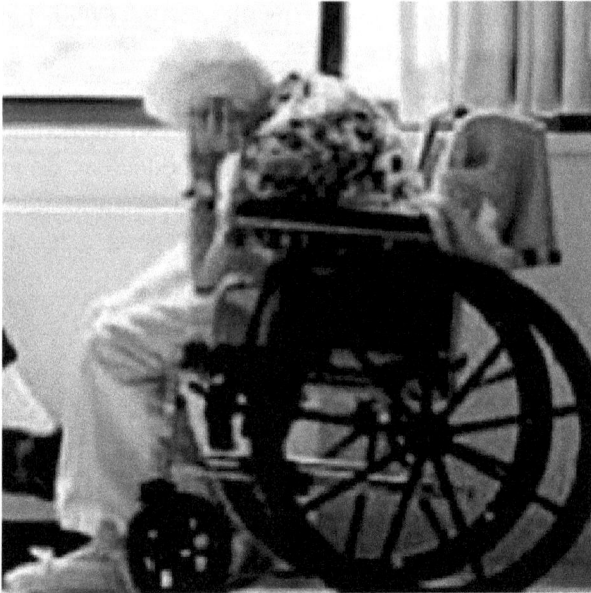

This lady does not look comfortable. She obviously wants something to lay her head against. The best she can figure out is to lean on her hand. Another form of torture by leaving a person in a wheel chair without reclining and without a headrest for long periods of time.

Best Wheelchairs For Those With Paralysis

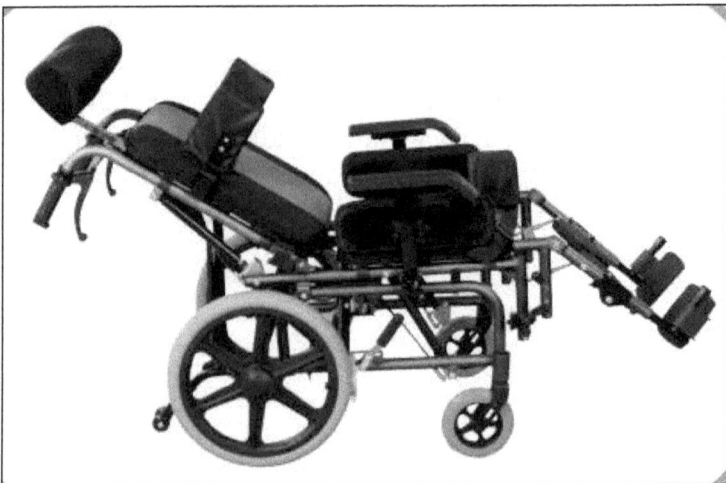

This model can sit up or recline: "Viper Plus Reclining with Flip Back Desk Arms-16." The Viper Plus Reclining is a reclining manual wheelchair with Flip Back desk arms for easy transfer, elevating leg rests for added patient comfort, push to lock wheel locks and "flip-up" anti-tippers with wheels. This Viper Plus model has a 16 inch seat width and a Weight capacity of 300 lbs. (other seat widths are available).

Other Features: Nylon padded armrests provide added patient comfort. New state-of-the-art hydraulic reclining mechanism. Front caster forks are adjustable in three positions.

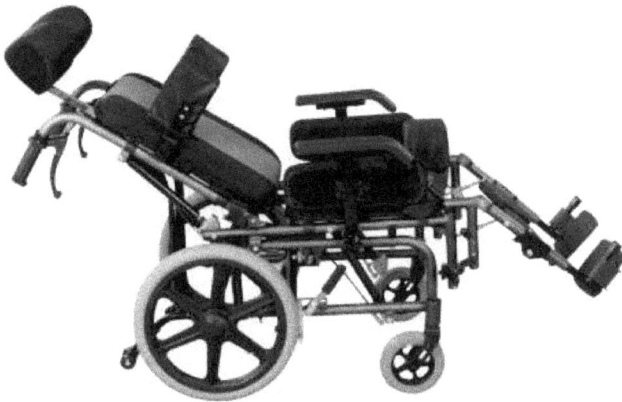

A simpler wheelchair with head rest and reclining back.

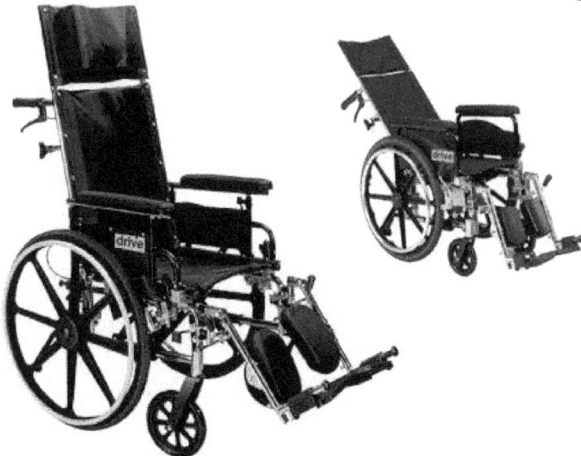

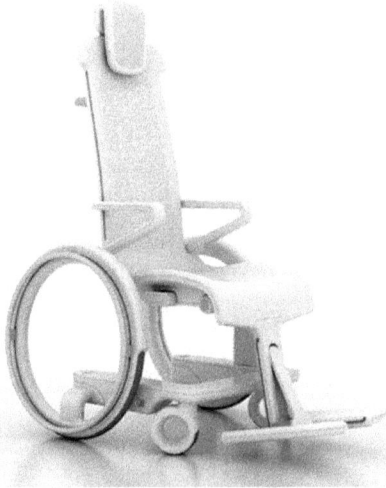

Home care chair

Wheelchair designed by Christen Halter adjusts to work in an upright, sitting and lying down position. The chair has a four wheel base and feet rests that fold up into the seat. Large wheels with hand grips can be added on to give the user the ability to propel themselves. The chair can be detached from its base and used on a stair-lift. The chair is made of high-tech materials for comfort and adjustable to suit the user's position.

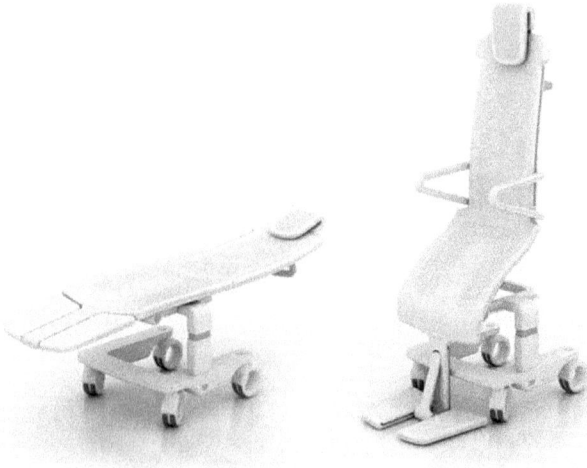

Classic Design Wheelchair

Designer David Pompa created these classic wheelchair designs as part of his inclusive objects series. Pompa questions why design icons are predominantly for an exclusive range of our society. To tackle this issue he added wheelchair wheels to a number of antiques and design classics like the lounge chair by Ray and Charles Eames. While the design is only a concept, it makes you think about the design of chairs versus that of wheelchairs. *[Author note: This might just be a prototype as I don't understand what keeps this designer office/house wheelchair from tipping over backward. MJW]*

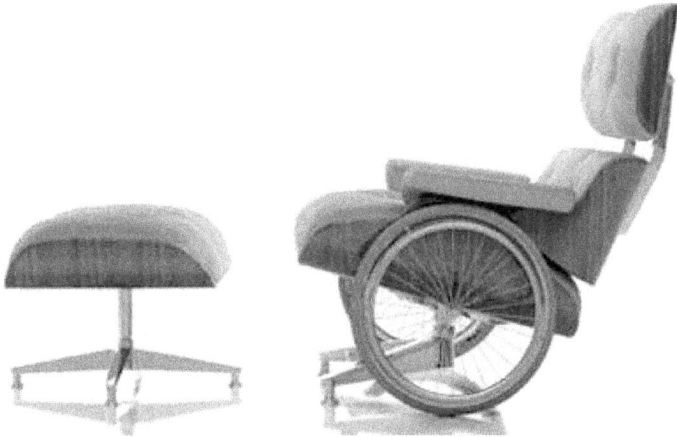

Wheelchair Bikes

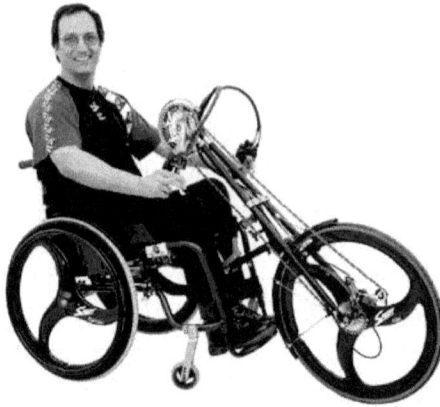

Speedy Bikes produces very special bikes designed to extend the function of wheelchairs. the company offers a range of wheelchair accessories that turn any wheelchair into a bicycle. Their designs simply attach onto regular wheelchairs and provide a method for propulsion through either foot pedals or hand pedals. But if pedaling around is too much trouble, they even have a device that transforms the wheelchair into an electric bike. The company also makes a low riding hand bike and an accessory for attaching to a regular bicycle to create a tandem bike.

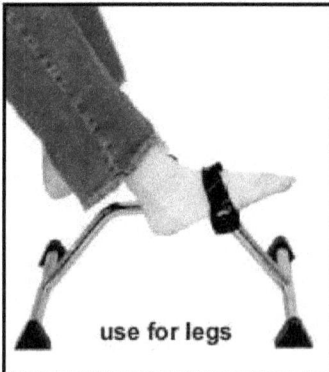

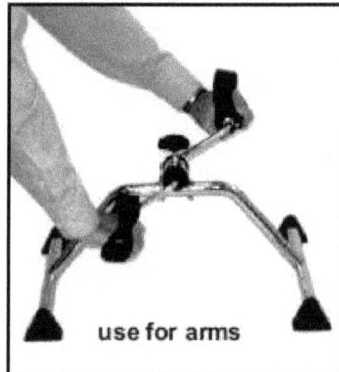

use for legs   use for arms

Leg and arm exerciser. The stronger limb can propel the weak or paralyzed side for nerve stimulation and improve blood flow.

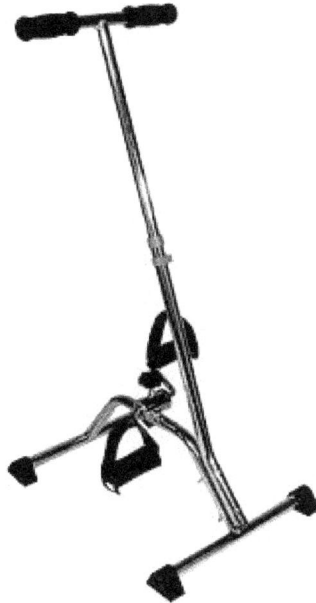

This Exercise Peddler with handle Stimulates circulation, ideal for toning leg muscles. The handle provides added stability while using Peddler and handle can be removed easily for storage. This exercise peddler with handle offers a Safe and gentle form of low impact exercise, often used for exercises for both elderly and stroke victims. The passive foot/leg will receive stimulation and motion through action of the active leg.

The next picture shows a grip to be suspended over the partially-paralyzed person's bed. They would be able to grab it with their mobile hand for their own exercise plus to be able to raise and move their shoulder on their non-paralyzed side.

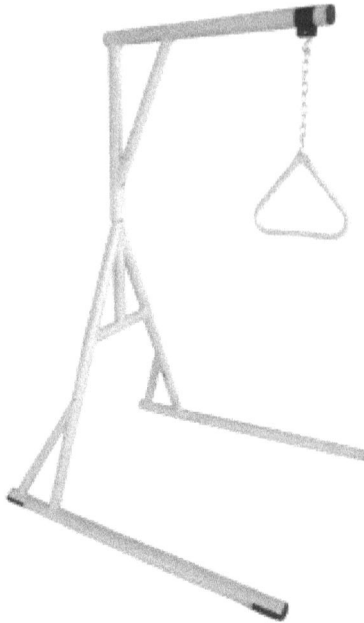

[Steve Hatch showed his visitors how handy and fun it was to use one of these suspended grips during his initial 16-day hospital stay after his stroke. When he recognized a visitor entering the Stroke rehab ward where he was located in the 4-bed ward, he would first shake their hand, then hold onto and show them the grip using his functioning hand. MJW]

I have not included the more common accessories like shower and tub seats, canes, and mobility seat/walkers. You probably see a lot of those in use for unstable persons. I'm just trying to disclose in this book the newer or recently invented handicapped items that might be perfect for someone with paralysis.

Don't forget, there are also automobiles designed for wheel-chair bound persons that can be driven with only their hand(s) and can include a wheel-chair lift to be operated by the disabled person alone. *[I will not include handicapped vehicles in this book as they are relatively common and must be adapted for each individual – in other words, one size does not fit all. MJW]*

Portable and Foldable Lift

The Molift Smart 150 Patient Lift can perform almost any patient movement or transfer tasks in even the most restricted areas. The lifting height is generous enough to simplify any lifting task, even lifting from the floor. Each Molift Smart 150 Patient Lift has a standard four-point suspension that can be used with a wide range of patient slings from Molift. Choose this lift for optimal safety, comfort, and longevity, with complete support and dignity.

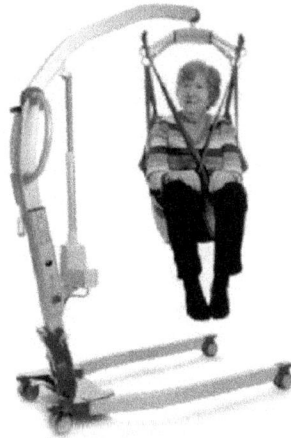

Arm and Leg Sling/Brace

Adjustable elbow brace for paralyzed arm. Correction brace for adults and children, one of assorted Orthotics tools. This brace helps keep their arm situated in a natural, comfortable position.

While sitting or lying down, support the paralyzed arm on an armrest or pillow to relieve shoulder pain from the arm's weight; the same should be done with a sling while walking. *[Many paralyzed people accidentally have their arm socket dislocated when being repositioned by their caregiver. They have absolutely no ability to tighten their shoulder muscles to prevent the arm from being dislocated at the shoulder so special care is needed by the person moving them.. MJW]*

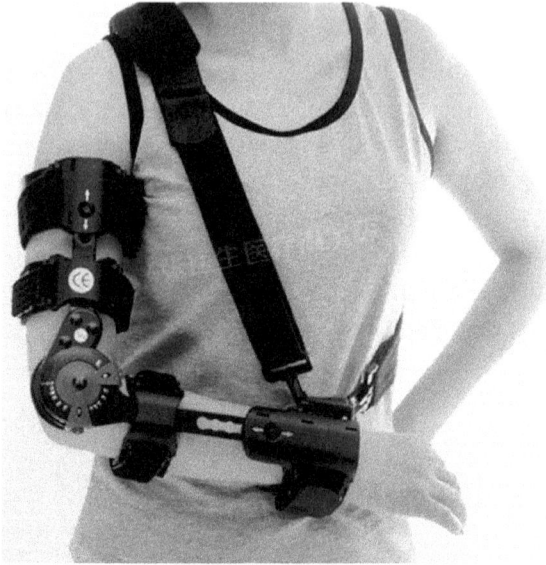

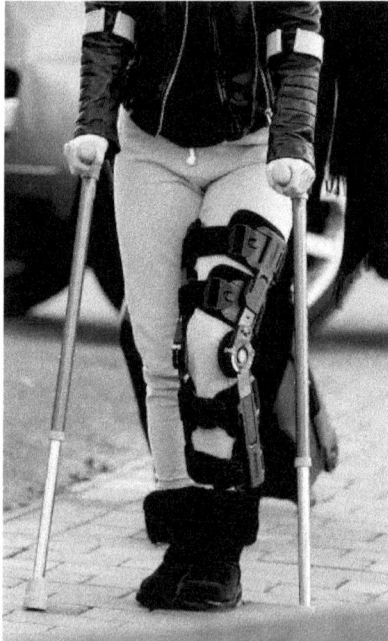

Leg brace to stabilize weakened/paralyzed muscles.

Most patients who have survived a stroke will have one leg that is paralyzed. This means that they cannot control the knee or ankle, but they are often able to control the hip. Since the ankle is essentially "floppy," the foot can get caught on each step and trip the survivor. Doctors refer to this phenomenon as foot drop. A prosthetic brace is often used called a foot-ankle-knee prosthetic. The equipment keeps the leg rigid and often allows for a stable base of support, despite the lack of movement in the leg. If the survivor can ambulate with this device, they may only need a cane.

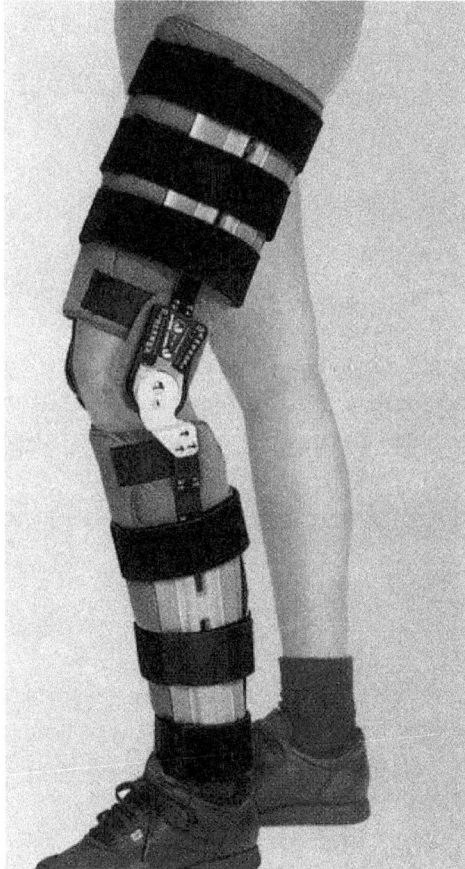

A leg brace.

For lower body dressing, you should put your brace on beforehand with the non-effected hand. Pull the leg over the paralyzed leg first. Then pull the non-effected leg into the other opening. You can even get equipment that helps you put on socks independently. It is a cupped piece of almost cylindrical plastic with a rope loop on the end. You put the sock over the end of the plastic, put your foot in the sock, and then pull the rope until the sock drifts over your heel. Many stroke survivors can also tie their shoes one handed, and it isn't as hard as it looks.

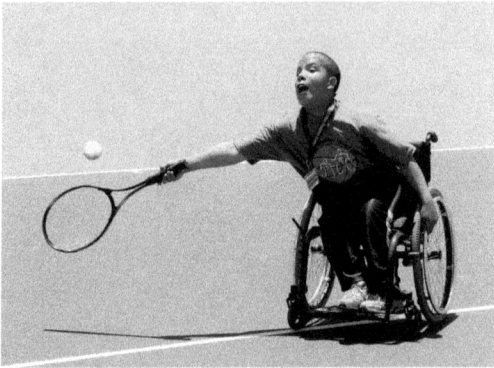

⮫Examples of sport wheelchairs. They are made for all ages and can be used for tennis, basketball and other team sports played in gymnasiums or on hard-surface outdoor courts.

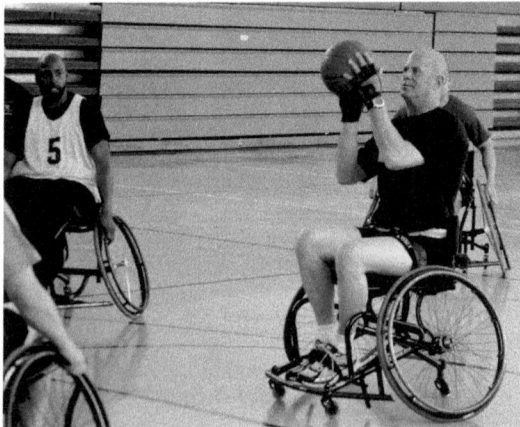

Exercise Equipment for Paralyzed People

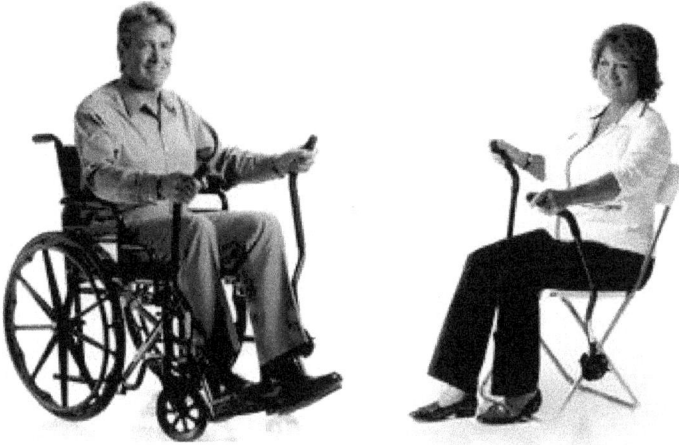

The Wheelchair Workout Exerciser accessory attaches to any wheelchair or chair to provide a cardio and upper-body workout from a seated position. Tone your abs and arms, engage your core, and lose weight/inches. Great for range of motion and the heart. Adjustable resistance to customize your workout. Great for stroke recovery, obesity, diabetes, balance issues, arthritis, geriatrics and many more. Comes fully assembled and easily attaches to your own chair or wheelchair

Handicapped Equipment for the Adventurer

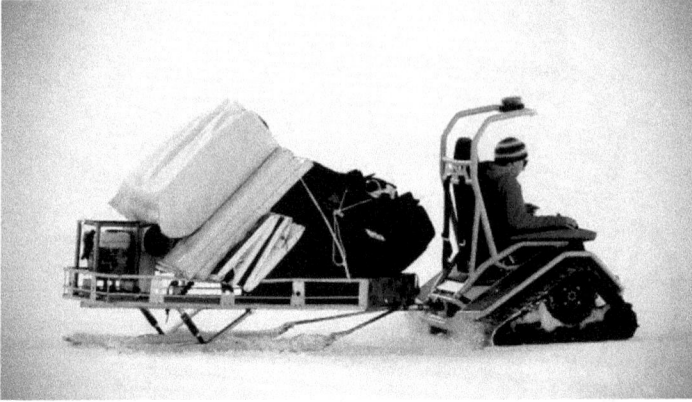

Handicapped winter explorer towing his gear using
a track-style motorized vehicle.

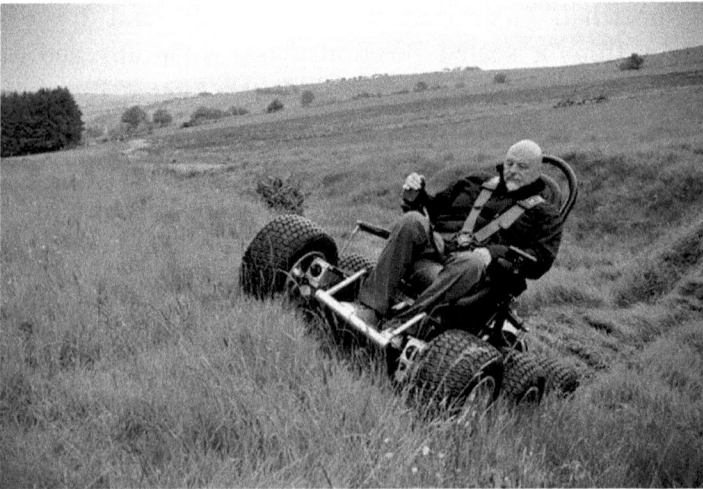

Climb hills with a powered 6-wheel vehicle
designed for the handicapped person.

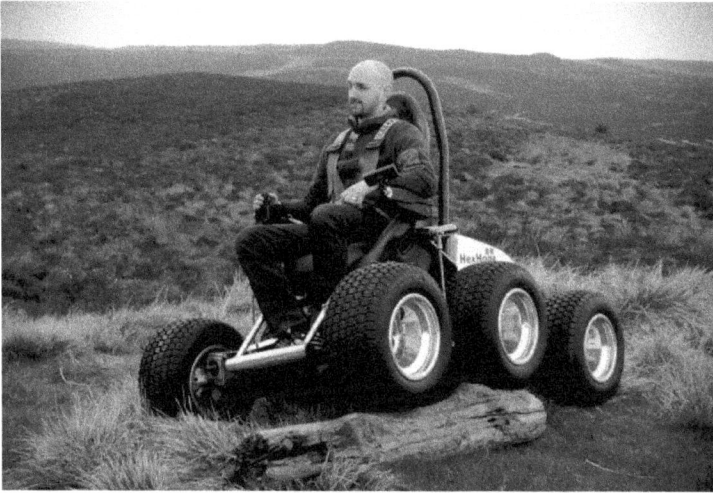

There is life after stroke.

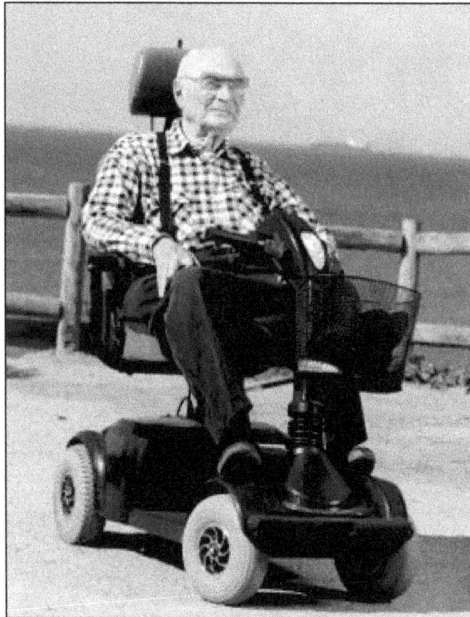

This man looks quite content with his motor vehicle. Since it has duel handlebars, he probably is not paralyzed in his arms, just not able to walk far. He has a head rest.

The Ultimate Stair Climber

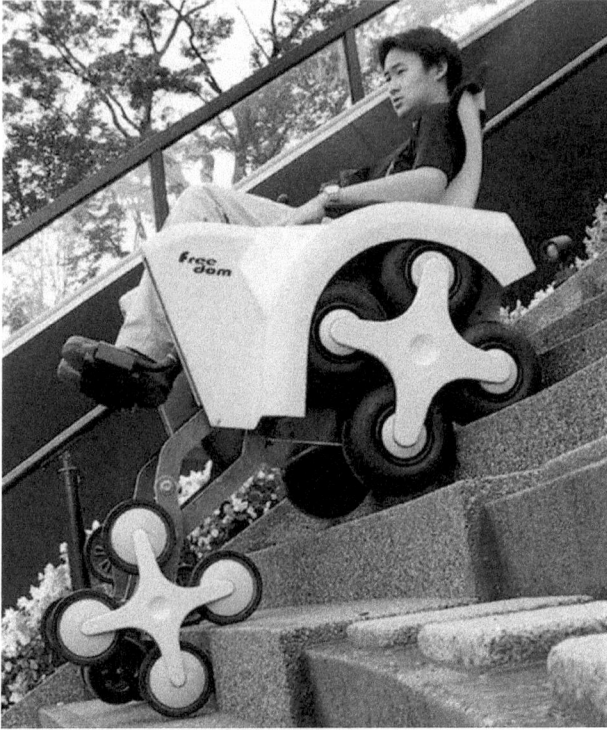

Going up and down stairs? No problem.

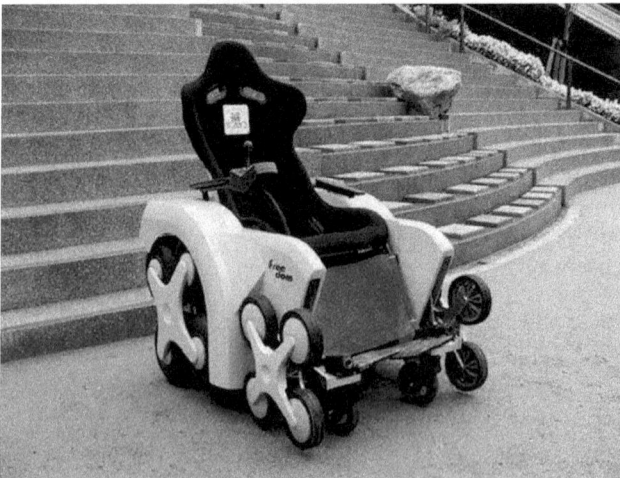

More stair-climbing machines.

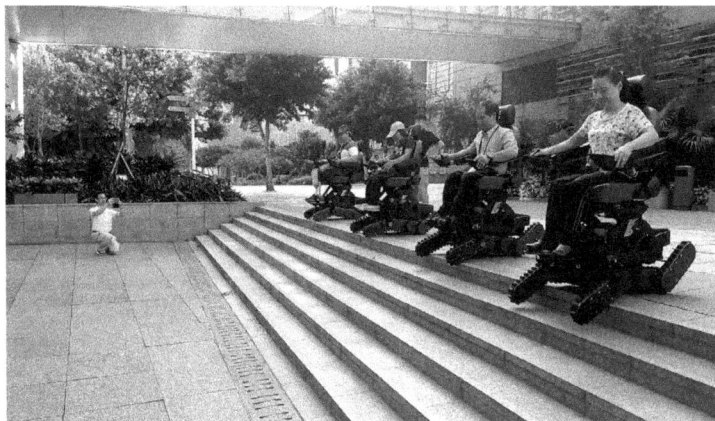

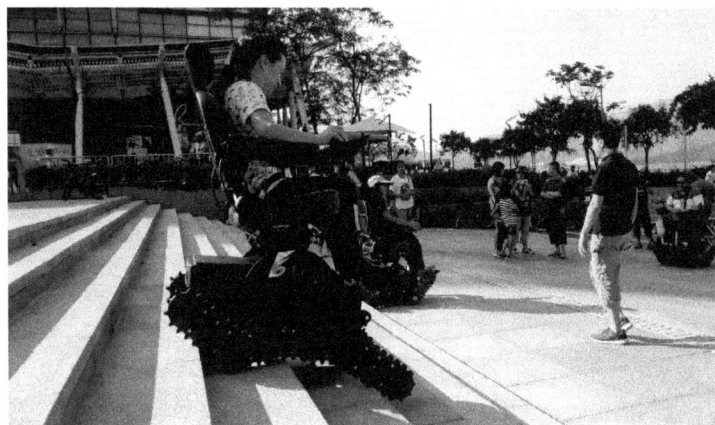

Electric Scooter for Handicapped Person
4 Wheel Scooter with 20" Captain's Seat

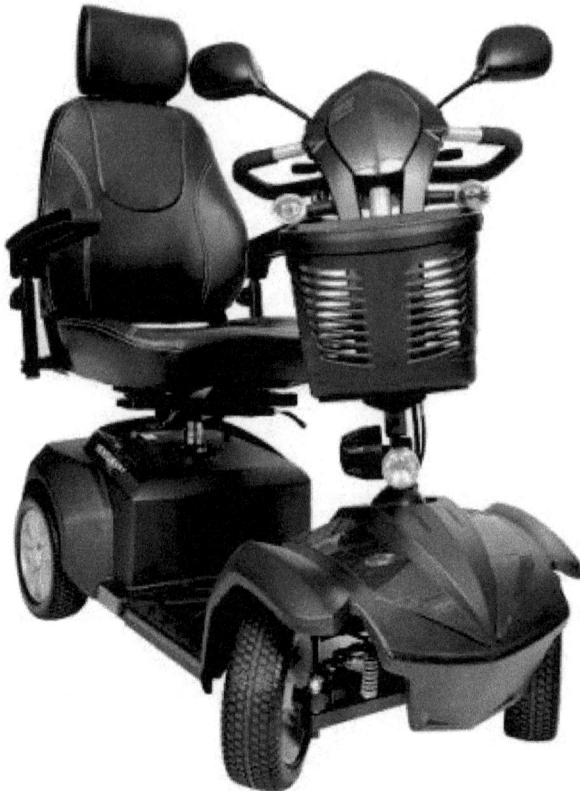

This scooter combines attractive styling with added comfort. The Ventura Dlx features a roomy 20 inch width captain's seat, the height-adjustable swivel seat features a fold-down backrest. The seat back reclines and has an adjustable headrest. The seat position can be adjusted forward and backward. The weight capacity is 350 lbs. *[Author recommends 4-wheeler for added tipping stability instead of 3-wheeler models. Also note the head rest which I endorse. MJW]*

Schedule and Goals for the Stroke Victim

The goal of stroke rehabilitation is to restore as much independence as possible by improving physical, mental and emotional functions. This must be done in a way that preserves your dignity and motivates you to re-learn basic skills that the stroke may have affected, such as eating, dressing and walking.

Rehabilitation should start in the hospital, as soon as possible after the stroke. If you are medically stable, rehabilitation may begin within one day after the stroke, and should be continued after release from the hospital, if needed. For others, rehabilitation can take place months or years later as your condition improves, or in some cases, worsens.

Stroke rehabilitation options will depend on several factors, including ability to tolerate intensity of rehabilitation (hours/stamina), degree of disability, available funding, insurance coverage, and your geographical area.

Stroke and Language Timeline

The ability to communicate through speech and gesture is something most people take for granted. From an early age, much of our life is dedicated to first acquiring, then exercising the natural skill of language as we conduct our family and business affairs.

Imagine suddenly losing the ability to order a restaurant meal, read the paper, understand a radio broadcast, or respond when spoken to.

For a stroke victim, at a time when he or she is already disoriented and afraid, the loss or impairment of language is a cruel blow. When brain tissue is damaged by a stroke, aphasia is the result in about 20 percent of stroke victims. Each aphasic person has a unique set of speech and language problems, accompanied by other symptoms caused by the same stroke.

Aphasia Timeline

Aphasia is marked by speech and language problems caused by damage to the brain. People with aphasia may have problems speaking, understanding speech, reading and writing (just one or all of these areas may be affected), ranging from mild to severe in nature. Aphasia does not generally affect the ability to think, reason and understand. Most aphasics know what they want to say - they just have trouble putting their thoughts into words. A similar inability to understand non-verbal forms of communication such as gestures and facial expressions may also exist.

Aphasia can take many forms. Some aphasics have word-finding difficulties (anomia). Some can only respond to a question by repeating it back, parrot-like (echolalia). Others use invented words (neologisms), or get "stuck" on a certain word, repeating it over and over (perseveration). Paraphasic errors, in which "dye" may be substituted for "tie" and/or "wife" for "husband" are also common.

Those with aphasia may have a grammar which is rational and orderly even though the words make no sense (fluent aphasia), or may use a word or two appropriately, but not produce meaningful sentences (nonfluent aphasia).

Dysarthria is a weakness or paralysis of the muscles of the face, mouth, neck and/or throat caused by brain injury, that may cause difficulties in talking, eating, swallowing and/or breathing, and cause speech to be slurred and sometimes unintelligible. It may occur with or without aphasia.

Aphasia does not get worse over time. Unless new brain damage occurs, almost all aphasic patients improve their use of language over time.

Speech Therapy Timeline

The speech / language pathologist assists the stroke patient in relearning the communication skills necessary to rejoin his or her family, friends, and colleagues. Intensive (four or five times weekly) speech therapy in the hospital setting usually begins soon after the patient is well enough to begin treatment. Generally, recovery is most likely to occur from three to six months after the stroke, plateauing after this period. However, improvement may continue for an indefinite period, depending on the patient's health, age, motivation, and the severity of the stroke.

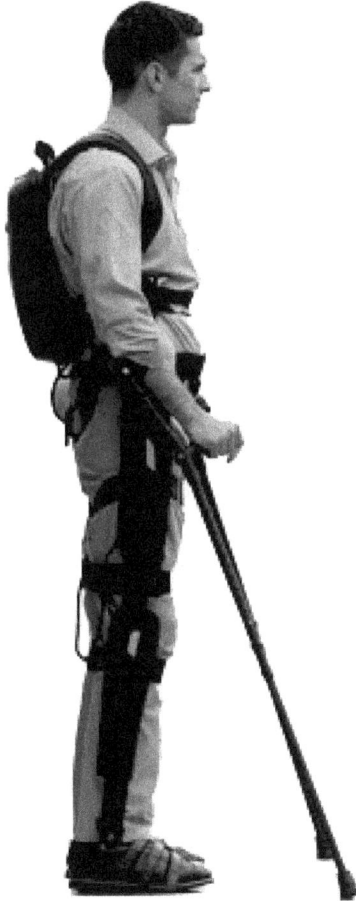

🐾Leg-brace allows man to walk with arm-crutches.

Aiding Recovery

While in the hospital

To maximize the patient's comfort and support his or her abilities, bring glasses, hearing aid and batteries, dentures and dental adhesives if needed.

Display clearly labeled photos of family and friends to help orient the patient.

Consult with the speech pathologist (or neurologist, case doctor and nurses in smaller hospitals) and ask what you can do. Comforting and communicating will be most successful if you understand your loved one's aphasia.

Don't assume that the aphasic person can't understand what's being said. Never say anything you wouldn't want the aphasic person to completely understand.

It is best to remember that the frustration of aphasia may cause irritability. It is normal to expect depression due to illness and stress in an aphasic stroke survivor, and chemical changes caused by stroke may result in deeper depression and apathy. The aphasic person (and stroke survivors in general) may not seem like the person you used to know.

Aphasia does not get worse over time. Unless new brain damage occurs, almost all aphasic patients improve their use of language over time.

On Returning Home for the Aphasic Person

Set up a daily routine for the aphasic person, being sure to provide rest periods - stroke survivors tire easily. Encourage both favorite and independent activities.

Aphasia is a family illness - support for the caregiver is as important as help for the aphasic person. Join a stroke support group. SRC provides peer support, fellowship, and helpful information to stroke survivors and their families.

Speech and Comprehension Aids

[Note: Author has not tested nor used any devices or apps found in this section. I merely want to give you a sampling of what is available. Also, the apps for your electronic devices come in full color, this book displays them in black/white. MJW]

Just using cardboard posters approximately a foot square with purchased signs or your own designs give the stroke victim symbols to point out their wants. Remember their eyesight may be affected for awhile so start out with large, simple symbols/characters.

Some people are also not able to read yet due to their brain mixing up words. Be patient, there will be something on a board they understand if you point to a food symbol and say "hungry?" They will soon get the connection and be able to associate spoken words to the corresponding symbol – and eventually even relearn the written word that corresponds to the symbol.

In the meantime, your ability to recognize eye movement or limited facial expressions of your loved one will also help indicate if you are getting close to the right question/need. You are the best judge of what your person is trying to say. True friends/loved ones often don't need words to communicate – eye contact says it all.

Follows are a sampling of some simpler cards that might be used for the first few weeks when speech is temporarily unavailable.

YES	NO

RESTROOM	HUNGRY	THIRSTY

Thank You	Please keep trying	1	2	3
YES	NO	NOT SURE	PEN PAPER	4	5	6
				7	8	9
				0		

A	B	C	D	E	F	G	H	I
J	K	L	M	N	O	P	Q	R
S	T	U	V	W	X	Y	Z	

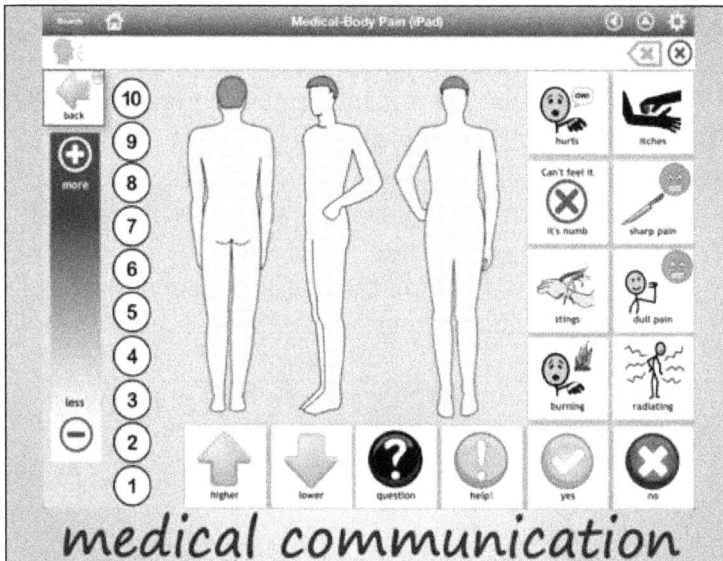

medical communication

To Aid Speech and Comprehension

- Speak slowly and clearly rather than loudly.
- Speak in clear, simple language. Face the person to allow them to see your mouth and facial expression - it will help them understand what you are saying.
- Encourage the aphasic individual to speak by engaging in conversation on a level they can handle. Look at pictures and photographs and discuss them. Help with word finding if they get stuck, but first allow them to try for themselves.
- Listen carefully and patiently, even if the person's speech is hard to understand. Complement them on their progress, no matter how small.
- Don't be condescending. Treat the aphasic person like the mature adult they are.
- One on one conversation is easiest for an aphasic person - two or more people speaking at the same time can be confusing and make comprehension impossible.

- If difficulties are experienced in reading, books with plenty of pictures or large print books may aid comprehension. Try reading your newspaper's weekend comics (the pictures help), then go on from there.
- Encourage stroke survivors to try to write and draw. If the dominant arm is impaired, stroke survivors should practice writing with their other hand. It may be easier to print before writing, and using large letters may help. If their hand is unable to grip a pen/pencil, there are holders to help.

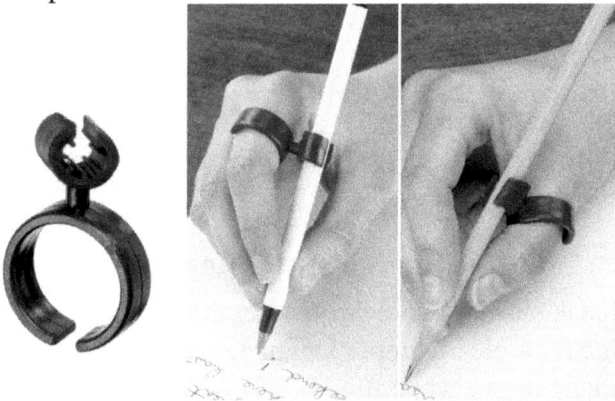

- In some cases, where writing and natural speech are not functional, alternative forms of communication must be explored, using adaptations and other strategies such as a communication board.

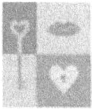

**How To Communicate
With Someone You Love:
Your Keys To Success**

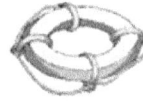

	Take time to communicate.
	Speak at a slow, normal rate.
	Talk in a quiet place.
	Write key words. Use pictures and drawings.
	Act it out.
	If it's not working, try another approach.
	Make sure you are on the same page.

Touch-Screen-Communication-Devices-for-Aphasia

- There are computerized stand alone devices. A keyboard is not important because many patients have the same problems trying to spell as trying to speak.
- An app for children but works brilliantly for simple interactions is called "Grace App." You can put it on an iPod Touch. You can edit and add items so you can set

your loved one up with a mouth icon on her home screen which they can literally touch to explain their condition.

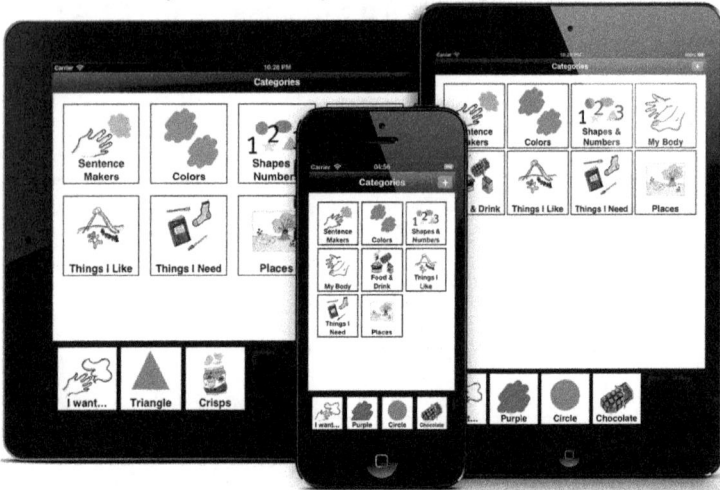

- A speech-language pathologist who works primarily with adults with aphasia suggests you may want to look at Proloquo2Go for the iPad. The app uses stick-figure icons but it is possible to add your own photos to the images library.

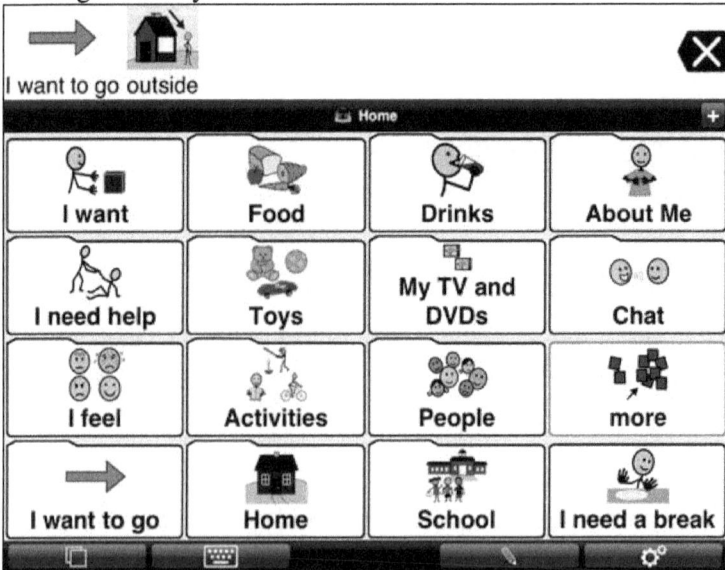

- Another device is called TouchTalk by Lingraphica for a variety of devices/computers.

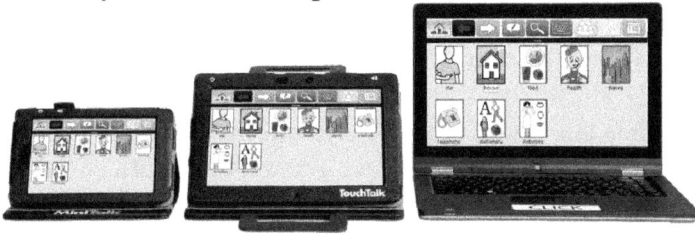

- A speech-language pathologist should be able to customize any app-based device without any specialized training. This should be done during the patient's treatment sessions with them as an active participant (i.e., no additional insurance billing beyond what's already being billed for that hour).

The most effective way to communicate is to ask simple closed questions in order of what your experience suggests is what the person might need and seeking a yes or no answer.

Another technique is using a sheet with yes / no written on it and you can track their eyes to get an answer. Remember that this is a frustrating time for them too and it may take a little longer than usual to find their answer.

The "TalkPath Speech Therapy Apps!" has updated reading, writing, listening, and speaking exercises. The apps are designed to help rebuild important speech-language skills for adults with aphasia. Additional features include:

- NEW CONTENT – Each app has a minimum of 800 exercises to help rebuild important speech-language skills like reading, writing, listening, and speaking. Some, like writing, have more than 1,500 exercises.
- USER-FRIENDLY – Your clients can select the difficulty level that best fits their needs.
- FUNCTIONALITY – Faster load times and redesigned cueing features.

You can also get the apps from iTunes

There are many other apps that will work with touch-screen apparatus for your loved one to use for communicating. You will find that once your person is able to make their simplest needs known to you (or the caregiver), they will be more relaxed. Follows are some screens from an assortment of apps. Author has not tested any of these but online searches can find many available and some which are very low-priced or free to download to your device.

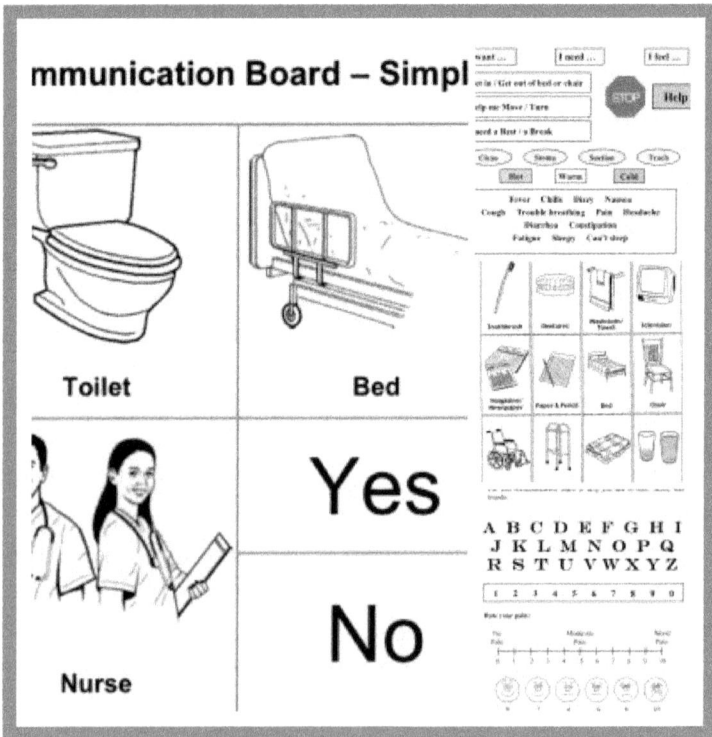

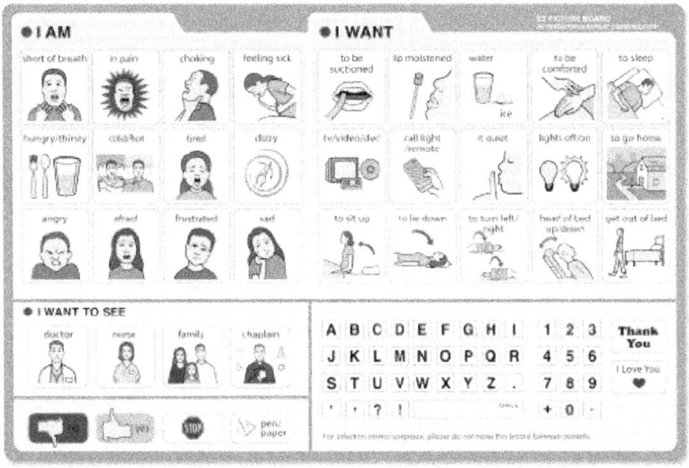
I AM
short of breath
in pain
choking
feeling sick
hungry/thirsty
cold/hot
tired
dizzy
angry
afraid
frustrated
sad
I WANT
to be suctioned
lip moistened
water
ice
to be comforted
to sleep
tv/video/dvd
call light /remote
lights off/on
to go home
to sit up
to lie down
to turn left/ right
head of bed up/down
get out of bed
I WANT TO SEE
doctor
family
chaplain
A B C D E F G H I
J K L M N O P Q R
S T U V W X Y Z .
1 2 3
4 5 6
7 8 9
+ 0
Thank You
I Love You
STOP
pen/ paper

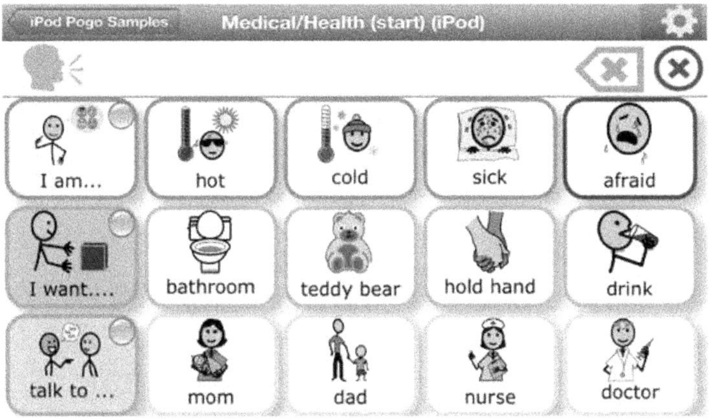
iPod Pogo Samples
Medical/Health (start) (iPod)
I am...
hot
cold
sick
afraid
I want....
bathroom
teddy bear
hold hand
drink
talk to ...
mom
dad
nurse
doctor

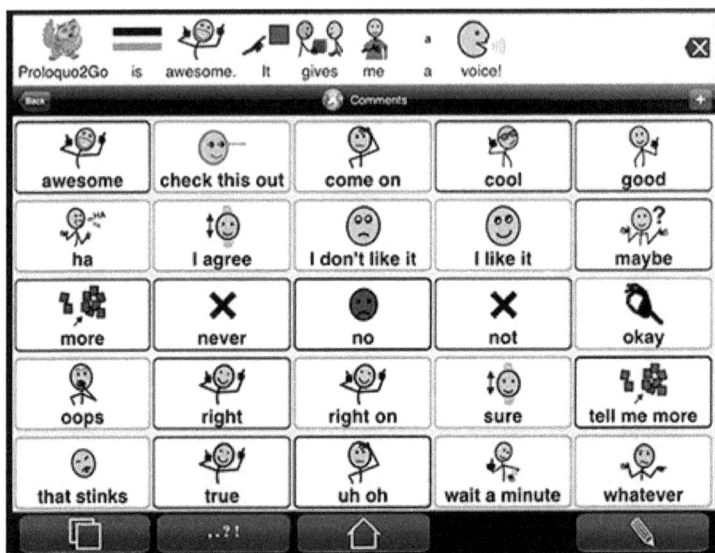

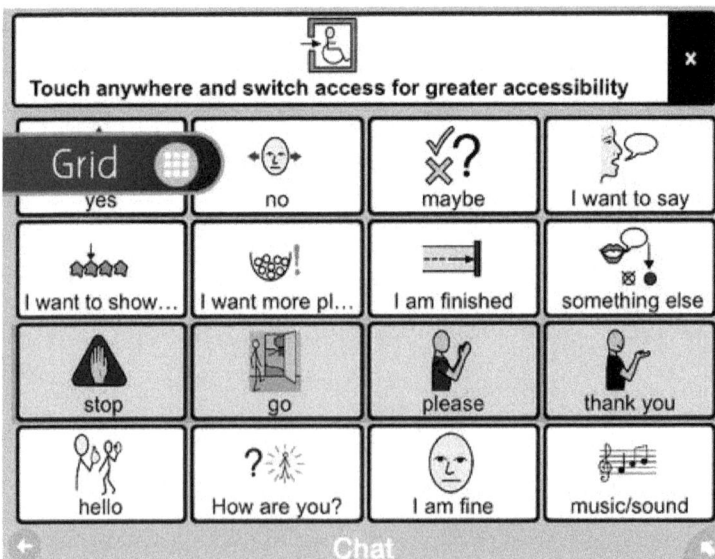

Meal Time

Depending on the stroke survivor, paralysis, one-sided weakness and/or dysphagia (trouble swallowing) can make feeding oneself difficult. Pay close attention to breathing and swallowing issues to avoid choking. Paralysis can also make it difficult for the stroke survivor to feed him/herself. Here are some suggested meal-time aids:

• Adaptive utensils with foam handles/grips.
• Plate guards.
• Cups with handles.
• Liquid thickeners

Follows are samples of utensils for those with weak or unsteady finger grip. People prefer to be as independent as possible. These examples of tableware include large, easy to grasp handles, bent angle for decreased wrist mobility, and thumb grip on spork (spoon/fork combination).

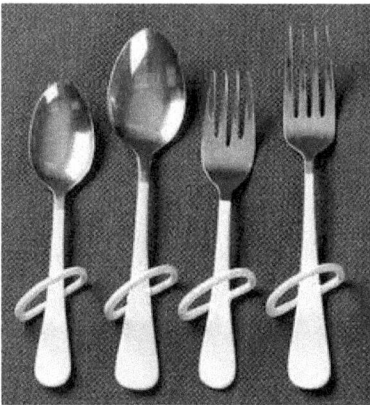

Left Hand Utensils

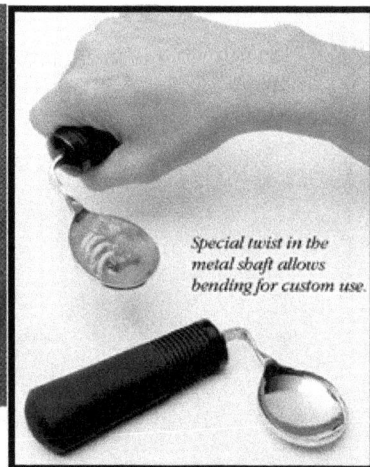

Special twist in the metal shaft allows bending for custom use.

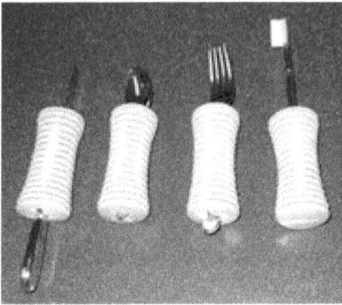
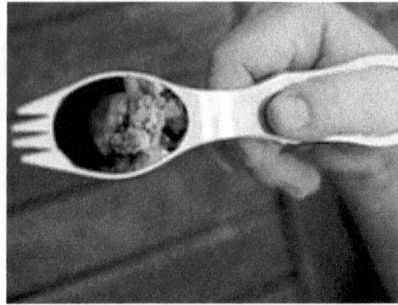

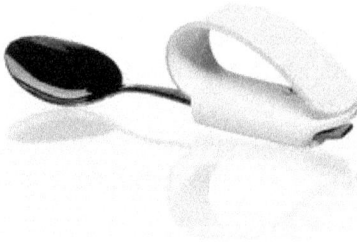
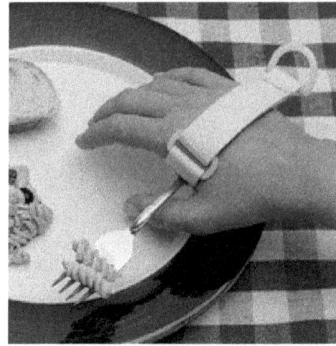

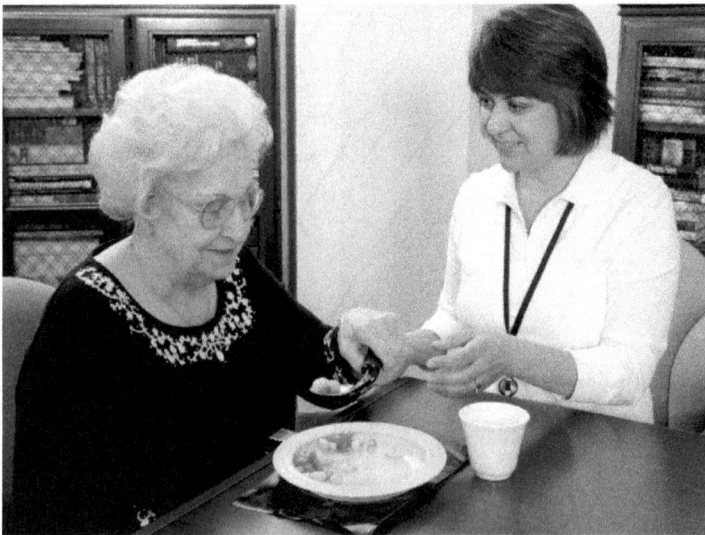

Activities For the Patient During Recovery

Computer and word games and puzzles will promote improvement (depending on the level of ability, children's learning tools can be very helpful).

Cognition (Thinking): Memory, attention span, self-awareness and comprehension skills may be diminished in a stroke survivor after the stroke. Your loved one may lose the ability to learn new tasks, remember things, problem-solve, understand things, make plans or acknowledge the reality of his/her physical limitations. There are a variety of ways to manage cognitive deficits as well as improve them:

- •Break up tasks into simple steps.
- •Set a routine.
- •Keep things the stroke survivor regularly uses (such as a toothbrush) in the same place.
- •Use prompts and reminders.
- •Repeat exercises.
- •Read.
- •Play card games, checkers, memory games, puzzles and crosswords to improve memory, focus and thinking skills.
- •Consult with a speech therapist and/or an occupational therapist for more exercises.
- Confinement (limited movement) If the stroke survivor is confined to a bed, move him/her often to protect against bed sores and skin irritations. Range-of-motion exercises and leg lifts will help with muscle strength, and installing bed rails is an essential safety feature. Safety monitors and walkie-talkies can also help you communicate with the stroke survivor when you are in another room.
- Make sure the confined person has a way to call you if they need something. One suggestion is one or more cowbells hung over the bed. It (they) must be accessible from multiple positions of the person no matter what side they are laying on. A series of cow bells (or similar bells)

could be suspended on chains near the head and along both sides of the bed. The larger the bell, the more noise it makes when it is tapped. It wouldn't hurt to have a couple near the foot where a swinging leg could reach them to call for assistance.

Remember, the completely bedfast person is worried they won't be able to get help in time if they are choking, or something is hurting, or their oxygen line has come loose and they are having trouble breathing. Just having some call-bells within reach will ease their anxiety.

The old-style cow bells were designed to hang from a horizontal leather strap and do not ring well if allowed to tip sideways where the gong is resting against the side. Some bells have rounded loops that automatically swing correctly.

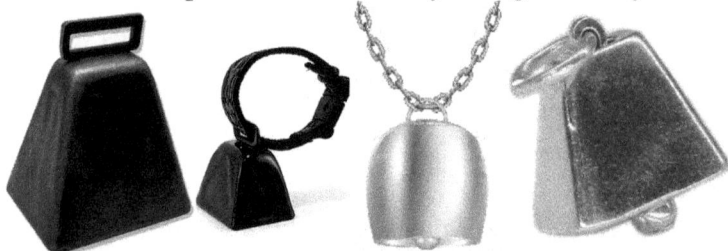

- There are other options for electric/electronic call-buttons but the majority of hospital buttons just lay on the bed and would be hard to find for a paralyzed person in the dark.
- Another possibility are infant's suspended crib toys that attach to the railing. They might be adaptable to hold noisemakers like bells or noisy toys.
- If you are really strapped for cash, you might be able to invent some noisemakers out of tin cans suspended across the head and/or foot of the bed to hit against each other and/or with gongs suspended inside.
- A series of large jingle bells might work

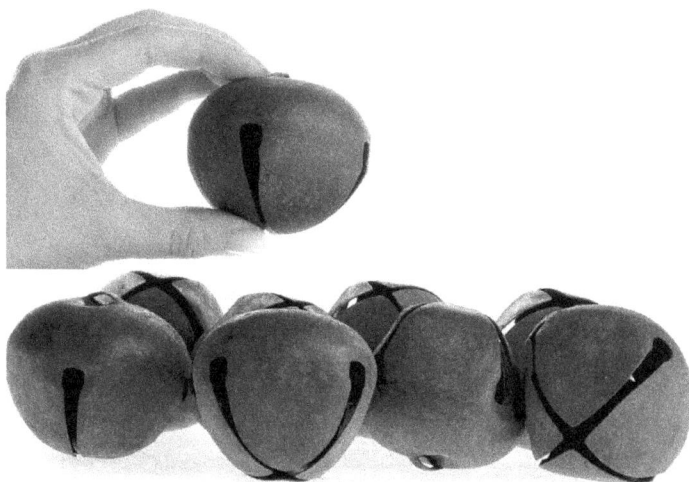

See the Home Modifications section for other safety suggestions including safety monitors to listen or to view someone in another room.

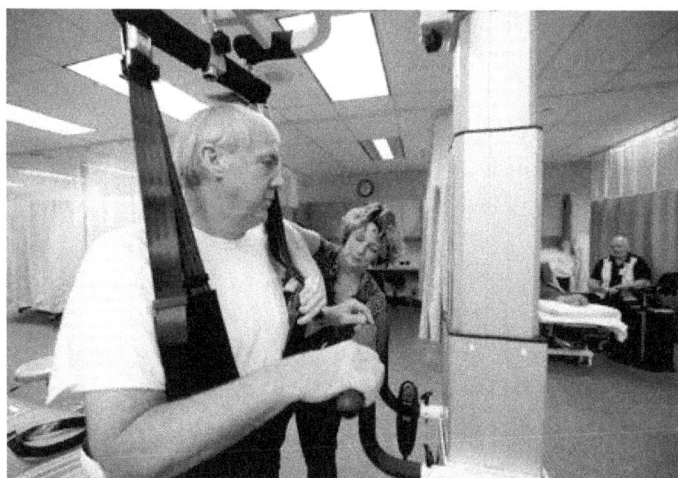

⇨Man being supported upright for therapy.

Funding Available Through Medicare

Medicare Home Health Care FAQ

What services are covered by Medicare for home health?

- Medicare requires a physician to write an order for home health services when medically necessary.
- The patient requiring services must be considered homebound during the time period services are ordered.
- With supporting diagnosis's, a patient may be able to receive skilled visiting nurse, physical therapy, occupational therapy, speech therapy, medical social worker and a home health aide to assist in bathing 2-3 times a week.

How do I pay for home care services through Medicare?

- Home health care agencies licensed to provide home care will not accept any money from you. Throughout the United States, there are a multitude of home health care agencies licensed to provide care and bill Medicare directly. The initial home health visit is done by a registered nurse.

Is there a co-pay or out of pocket expense I have to pay?

- There is no co-pay or out of pocket expense to receive Medicare home health.

When should I expect a visit by the home care agency?

- What is normal and customary is for the home health care clinical supervisor or intake coordinator to contact you the evening before or the morning of the visit. The nurse generally will give you a window of hours that they will be arriving to your home.

How often can I expect a visit from the home health care agency?

- Based on the ordering physician and medical needs, agencies will determine the frequency and duration of visits during the initial oasis evaluation conducted by the nurse the first home visit. For the most part, agencies will tend to stagger the visits with nursing on one day and therapy the following alternating days.

If the visiting nurse finds something medically wrong with my spouse, do I have to notify the doctor?

- It is the responsibly of the visiting home care nurse to notify the physician of the patient's condition. The doctor may adjust medication and provide additional orders to the agency in order to maximize care.

How long is a home health order good for?

- When a physician writes a prescription for home health services, the order is good for a 60 day period. Should additional care be required outside the 60 days, the home health care agency can request the physician for recertification to extend the visits.

What can I expect once my doctor orders Medicare Home Health Care Services?

- Whether you or a loved one experienced a recent health setback and is being discharged from a local hospital, a skilled nursing and rehabilitation facility or visited a primary care physician, it is customary to be notified by the home health care agency within 24 to 48 hours. The doctor writes an order for a home health evaluation so the nurse can become the eyes and ears for the doctor. Home health service is designed so that patients can heal in the comforts of their own home and not in a hospital or skilled nursing and rehabilitation bed.

- Medicare home health is important especially during the transition of care. Should an order derive from a skilled nursing and rehabilitation center or from a hospital stay, the discharge paperwork will have written the home care agency's telephone number. A Medicare patient or caregiver can expect to receive a call regarding the visit setting an appointment time. It is advised if possible the caregiver be available during the initial home visit so that realistic expectations of duties covered by Medicare are explained as well as a review of the medication. The nurse will assess and review basic demographic information, document patient's ambulatory status, living situation, family and social support and assess safety in the home.

Who can order Medicare Home Health Services?

- Any licensed physician that is a Medical Doctor or DO can order home health care services for a patient within the same state. The doctor must also certify that the patient is under his/her care and have had a face to face encounter within the 90 days prior to the start of home health care or within the 30 days after the start of care with the patient.

Why is a face to face encounter required?

- Mandated by the Affordable Care Act (ACA), face to face paperwork completed by a physician is a mandatory condition for payment by Medicare to the home care agency. The face to face encounter is another way the Center of Medicare and Medicaid Services implements safeguards to make sure Medicare dollars are being used properly and not over utilized.

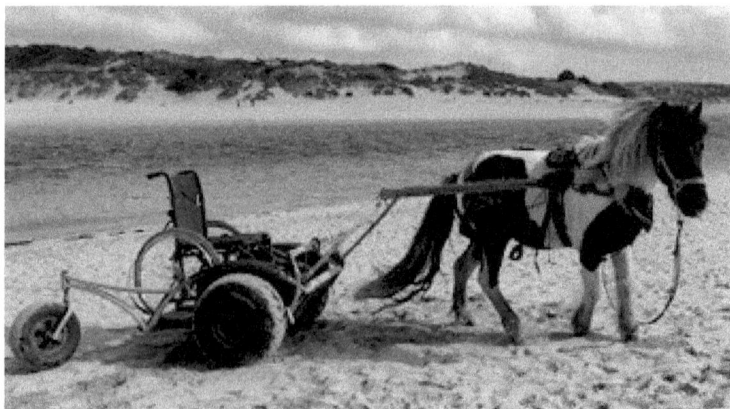

Pony-pulled beach wheelchair. Hitch has
quick release incase pony is startled.

Stroke Victims and Their Caregivers
Tips and Suggestions

Six Facts About A Person After A Stroke

I can still smell the flowers. I don't garden anymore, but I can still smell the flowers. Bring me some roses. This will remind me of my past.

I can still communicate. I can't talk the way I used to, but I can still communicate. Be patient as I try. This will help me feel connected.

I can still make decisions. I don't have the judgment I used to, but I can still make decisions. Give me choices. This will make me feel like I'm a part of things.

I can still wash my face. I can't take a bath by myself anymore, but I can still wash my face. Assist me with direction. This will help me feel purpose.

I can still sing. I can't dance anymore, but I can still sing. Help me enjoy music. This will enrich my life.

I can still move my body. I can't walk unassisted anymore, but I can still move my body. Walk with me, and support me if I stumble. This well help me feel engaged.

You are my lifeline. I depend on you. But please don't do for me what I can do for myself. Recognize what I can do and help me to function as a person.

You are key to the quality of my life.

Caregiving Guide: Caring for Yourself
and a Stroke Survivor

The rehab care team is involved in facilitating the stroke survivor's post-stroke recovery therapy. These experienced professionals specialize in rehab.

Case manager/Social Worker: Involved in discharge planning, coordination of services and connecting stroke survivors with local resources.

Occupational therapist (ot) Works with stroke survivors to regain skills for daily living activities and increased independence.

Physiatrist Specializes in rehab therapy and helps determine appropriate treatment plans to manage pain and disabilities involving muscles, nerves and bones.

Physical Therapist (PT) Engages stroke survivors in exercise techniques to increase mobility, reduce pain, prevent disability and restore independent functioning.

Social Worker May be involved in discharge planning, continuing care and connecting stroke survivors with resources.

Speech Therapist (ST) Works with stroke survivors with aphasia and apraxia issues to regain and improve language skills.

Vocational Therapist Assists stroke survivors who want to return to work, volunteering and other social activities.

The Primary Care Provider (PCP) usually provides the prescriptions for ongoing rehab therapy. Ask whether rehab should be part of your stroke survivor's recovery because it is not always necessary. It may be necessary to contact your insurance representative to find out what your benefits package covers.

The Rehab Care Team will begin rehab as soon as it is prescribed by the ordering physician. Rehab is essential in helping stroke survivors regain independence and life skills. While rehab does not cure a stroke survivor or completely repair damage to brain tissue, it can help a stroke survivor regain skills and promote recovery.

Look into specific stroke-certified rehab centers through the Joint Commission on Accreditation of Healthcare Organizations (TJC) and the Commission on Accreditation of Rehabilitation Facilities (CARF). TJC evaluates healthcare facilities and programs on their care and certifies those that meet all industry standards for safety, accountability and quality. CARF certifies stroke rehab facilities to ensure they are comprehensive, person-centered and use best practices in their care.

Home Modifications

Home modifications may be necessary depending on the stroke survivor's needs. Making appropriate modifications will enable the stroke survivor to regain independence throughout recovery. If facing financial challenges, be creative and seek help with your home modifications from friends, neighbors, faith communities, veterans groups and community organizations. Look for stores and/or websites that sell affordable new/used adaptive equipment and medical supplies. Examples of home adaptation include:

•Installing ramps that can be built or purchased.

•Rearranging or removing excess furniture and rugs to avoid falls.

•Checking lighting to ensure that walkways are well lit and to determine whether current window coverings need to be changed.

•Modifying the kitchen to ensure safety and accessibility.

•Checking the stair and wall rails for sturdiness.

•Installing grab bars, shower chairs and raised toilets in the bathroom.

•Acquiring medical supplies and assistive living devices (e.g., gait belts, adaptive cups and utensils and safety monitors to listen to someone in another room).

•Determining whether an emergency alert device is necessary.

•Having a key for emergency access. Install a lockbox or leave a key with your neighbor. This avoids the need for personnel to knock down your door in case of emergency.

Respite Care

Throughout caregiving, remember that you have options. Respite care refers to short- term relief services for the stroke survivor so you, the caregiver, can take a break. Caregivers providing unpaid care are eligible for respite care under the 2006 Federal Lifespan and Respite Care Act. Online registries, newspapers and yellow pages can be helpful in finding respite providers, or ask your medical and rehab care team members if they can make a referral.

Paralysis and Muscle Weakness Therapy

Paralysis refers to a person's inability to move muscles voluntarily. When messages from the stroke survivor's brain to his/her muscles don't work properly after a stroke, a limb can become paralyzed or develop spasticity, which is when muscles become tight or stiff, restricting movement. Stiffness in the arms, fingers or legs, painful muscle spasms or a series of involuntary rhythmic muscle contractions and relaxations can lead to uncontrollable movement or jerking.

Upper and lower limb movement issues can make balance and coordination difficult increasing risk of falling. Paralysis and weakness disrupt movement affecting daily activities. There are therapies available to help relearn motor skills and strengthen the arms and legs. Many physical therapists recommend stretching, walking or range-of-motion exercises.

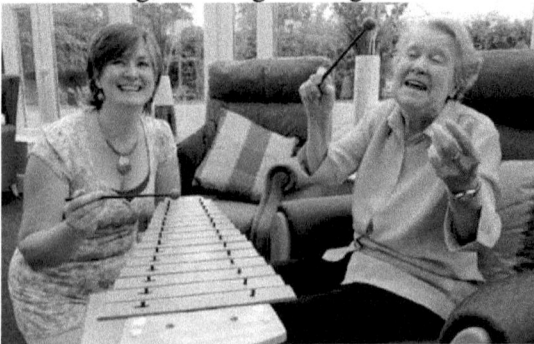

♬Music Therapy is fun for therapist and patient.

What to do if someone is having a seizure?

- Roll the person on his/her side to prevent choking or vomiting.
- . Cushion the person's head.
- Loosen any tight clothing around the neck.
- Keep the person's airway open. If necessary, grip the person's jaw gently and tilt his or her head back.
- Do not restrict the person from moving if he/she is in danger.
- Do not put anything in the person's mouth, not even medicine or liquid.
- Remove any sharp or solid objects that the person might hit during the seizure.
- Note how long the seizure lasts and what symptoms occurred in order to inform a doctor or emergency personnel if necessary.
- Stay with the person until the seizure ends.

Fatigue can make it difficult to perform daily tasks or stay motivated. Many stroke survivors report that they feel like they're "hitting a wall." Communication is vital to managing fatigue—ask the stroke survivor questions and encourage them to let you know when they feel tired.

- Physical fatigue —Motor deficits or muscle weakness and spasms.
- Cognitive fatigue —Memory loss, mental exhaustion and/or difficulty focusing.
- Emotional fatigue —Can co-exist with mood disorders, loss of motivation.

How to Prevent Recurrent Stroke

Alcohol: Reduce or eliminate alcohol consumption. Drinking more than two alcoholic drinks in one day raises a person's risk for stroke by 50 percent. Alcohol can negatively affect many organs and systems. Alcohol depresses the central nervous system and inhibits the liver's ability to produce proteins that regulate blood clotting. This thins the blood, which can be a good and a bad thing.

Alcohol also influences platelet (irregularly shaped cell fragments that circulate in the blood) function. Too many platelets cause excessive bleeding and too few cause blood clots. Alcohol contributes to platelet activation; activated platelets are more "sticky" than normal ones, causing blood clots. One drink of alcohol increases platelets a little, but excessive drinking causes too many platelets to activate, thus increasing risk for clots.

Over time, excessive alcohol use can lead to long-term increases. Alcoholic beverages usually contain a lot of calories as well, which can contribute to weight gain. The influence alcohol has on an individual depends on the person's age, gender, height, weight, genetics, level of hydration and medications. While some research says that drinking a small or moderate amount of alcohol can be beneficial in reducing risk of stroke, always consult with a healthcare professional. Heavy drinking can also increase the risk for atrial fibrillation in men.

Atrial fibrillation (Afib) is an irregular, rapid heartbeat that impairs a person's heart functioning because it slows blood to the heart. Afib is a major risk factor for stroke with no visible symptoms. A person with Afib is five times more likely to have a stroke. However, 75 percent of Afib-related strokes can be prevented with the use of anticoagulant medications that thin the blood. Because the risk of blood clots increases in those with Afib, anticoagulants are essential to prevention.

Diabetes is a group of chronic conditions where a person has high levels of sugar in the blood because of the body's inability to produce and/or use insulin. Medical treatment and dietary changes will be essential to manage diabetes, which increases the risk for stroke.

Exercise: Staying active and exercising for 30 minutes five times a week can help a stroke survivor stay healthy and reduce risk factors. Exercise doesn't necessarily mean walking, running or lifting weights. Talk to the stroke survivor's medical and rehab care teams for exercises that can be done at home.

High Cholesterol is a fat that is present in the outer layer of every cell in the body. It is produced by the liver and is necessary for normal bodily functioning. A cholesterol level of over 200 is considered high and raises the risk for recurrent stroke. High cholesterol can be caused by smoking, drinking too much alcohol, being overweight, not exercising and eating foods that are high in saturated fat. Medical treatments and diet changes are effective in lowering cholesterol. Talk with the stroke survivor's medical care team about appropriate treatment for high cholesterol.

Hypertension: High blood pressure, or hypertension, is another major risk factor for stroke. A blood pressure reading of 140/90 indicates hypertension. Talk with the stroke survivor's medical care team about effective strategies to lower blood pressure. Medical treatments, diet changes and exercise are most common.

Nutrition: Low-sodium, low-fat diets with lots of fruits and vegetables are best.

Stroke Survivor Guide – Activities to Entertain

You should look into computer games and those on tablets. Several   popular games, such as Candy Crush Saga and Bejeweled, only require that   you line up three symbols in a row.

Checkers

Listening to music or playing tunes on a portable piano keyboard with one hand.

Sculpting with soft clay is very therapeutic for contracted hands.

Most stroke survivors need a cane with four contact points for stability. This is called a quad cane.

Ambulatory Aids

Stroke survivors can use many different types of adaptive equipment for   ambulating. The most common is the simple cane. Although single point canes are usually what come to mind, most stroke survivors need a cane with four   contact points for stability. This is called a quad cane.

Walkers are another ambulatory aide that can be used. The determination between a cane and a walker can be tricky. It will depend on how much strength is left in the non- paralyzed leg and how stable a stroke survivor is on their feet. Walkers are for those who need a bit more help, but there are many types of walkers now that   can actually enhance lifestyle by substituting as a chair.

Dressing Equipment

Many adaptive devices are available to help stroke survivor dress   independently. With only one arm, it may seem impossible for them to dress themselves, but many do.

For instance, putting on a pull over shirt starts with putting the paralyzed arm into the sleeve first, pulling the shirt over the head, and   then putting the functioning hand through the remaining arm. With highly functioning stroke survivors, this is a skill they can perform with practice.

For shirts that are button up, there is a special loop that can help pull buttons through. You put on the shirt much like the pull over, then pull the two sides together. The button tool is a metal loop on the end of a stick. Push the metal end through the button hole, then loop it around the corresponding button. Simply pull it through. Again, this takes a good deal of practice.

Bathroom Modifications

The bathroom can be a dangerous place for stroke survivors, and this is where adaptive equipment is the most important to use. Grab rails are absolutely necessary in both the toilet area and the bathtub. They should be professionally installed on the studs to ensure that they are secure for the full weight of the stroke survivor. Usually, a contractor can help install these bars for a fee.

Another type of equipment is a raised toilet seat. It is a round piece of plastic that is about four inches in height. It has a hole in the center for the use of the toilet. The seat rests on the toilet with no further installation, and it can be removed easily.

For bathing, it may be hard to safely and independently perform this act as a stroke survivor. One piece of equipment that is needed is a shower chair. There are many different configurations of shower chairs, some that even come over the side of the tub to allow transferring from a wheelchair to the shower chair. It is important not to lean over too far while taking a shower. The survivor can easily pitch forward and suffer a head injury.

A simple sponge on the end of a stick can allow them to wash the parts of them they cannot reach with their hands. Again, stroke survivors should be monitored while bathing to ensure safety. Even if they are shy, the bathroom is a place of dangers that supersede any personal fears. Although they may not appreciate it, supervision is   absolutely necessary for bathing, but most of the washing itself can be done with adaptive equipment.

Although complete blindness is rare, partial blindness is one of the hallmark visual complications after a stroke. If you or your loved one had a stroke and are concerned over visual side effects, speak to your neurologist. They will be able to test visual fields to ensure that the eye and their corresponding nerves are working properly.

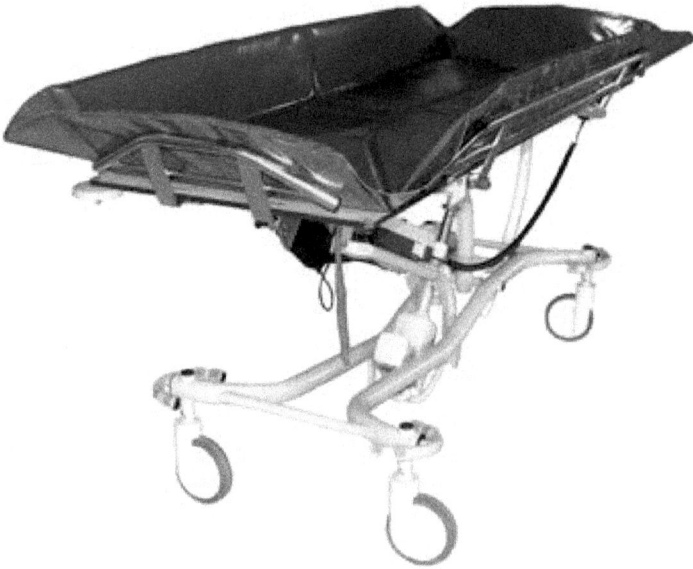

↰Portable bath carts can be used for sponge-baths without getting the bedding wet. Adjustable height makes transferring patient from bed to cart and back fairly simple.

Speech After Stroke – Technical Description

One of the most common symptoms of a stroke is slurred speech. Speech impairment coupled with numbness of the face or the extremities, visual impairment, dizziness and loss of coordination, and severe headache, calls for immediate medical attention.

A stroke is the interruption of blood flow to the brain, depriving brain cells from oxygen. These cells die after a few minutes, causing a loss of the neurological functions controlled by those cells. Strokes affecting the parietal lobe, Broca's center or Wernicke's center are likely to affect speech.

There are several types of speech difficulties which may arise after a stroke:

- Aphasia is an acquired language disorder affecting the ability to produce and understand language, as well as reading and writing.
- Dysarthria is a motor disorder affecting the control of speech muscles. Information transmitted to the tongue, throat or lips is disrupted, resulting in poor articulation.
- Apraxia of speech (or verbal apraxia) is the inability to produce information commanding speech muscles.

Treating Language Disorders

The goal of rehabilitation of speech impairments, is to restore a person's confidence in communicating with others. This may prove to be a difficult task, but people giving assistance should realize that the ordeal a stroke patient endures because of speech difficulties can be frustrating and should be met with a greater deal of patience and understanding.

Most patients with aphasia will have difficulty understanding words or expressing thoughts to words. Rehabilitation should be trained on understanding spoken language, making use of additional aids, if necessary. For example, one can use pictures which the patient can try to identify. This will help in recognition of several objects and translation of thoughts into words. Another exercise recommended is to give multiple clues leading to a word, stimulating the patient to think.

Patients may also be allowed, at first, to use hand gestures or signals to compensate for lack of appropriate words or just to help in carrying out a train of thought during a conversation. But, this should not let the patient and his therapist deviate from the ultimate goal of reestablishing the language capabilities. The hand gestures should only be used as an initial tool, so as not to contribute to the patient's frustrations.

It is important to keep in mind that together with rehabilitating the language capabilities, the patient's confidence needs nurturing as well.

The difference with this impairment is that the speaker is well aware of his mistakes, but still has difficulty in correcting them.

Apraxia therapy approaches include teaching sound production, rhythm and rate. Again, the exercises entailed in the therapy are aimed at practicing speech patterns, such that the brain sends out the necessary impulses to coordinate facial muscles for generating speech. Tasks may involve repetition of syllables and words to train the lips, mouth and tongue into making these sounds once again. Providing tips on proper placement of the tongue or shape of lips and mouth while producing sounds also helps in this therapy.

Dysarthria, on the other hand, leaves a patient struggling to move the speech muscles because they become too weak or too tight as a result of the stroke. Additional medical help from healthcare personnel should be heeded to identify the specific type of dysarthria, since it is crucial for the treatment. For example, strengthening exercises are appropriate when the muscles are weak, but may be harmful when the muscles have too much tone. A speech language pathologist should be able to aid in the identification and consequently recommend the proper therapy.

Usually, dysarthria rarely requires therapy and often disappears a few months after the stroke. But, in the event that the impairment persists, a more rigid therapy program may be suggested by the speech language pathologist.

Ultimately, the goal in the rehabilitation of stroke patients with speech difficulties should be to try and bring the patient to his normal, usual speaking self. This can only be achieved with providing the patient not just the therapeutic exercises but also with the environment that minimizes their frustration in having to re-learn common, everyday activities such as speech. This is very important in the recovery process, because speech does much in enabling the patient, making him a more independent and confident individual.

Exercises you can do to have unslurred speech: One of the exercises is to have an object identified in front of the patient – a label or repeating the name would help. Trying approving the patient's effort in communicating whether it is a gesture or little sounds. Encouragement is really helpful.

If the pronunciation is wrong, accept it. The patient was able to associate objects and names and this is part of the recovery process -- Baby steps.

Try avoiding set drills and exercise. Repetition has nothing to do with communicating. Vary each days exercises from time to time – like what food they want to eat, like clothes to wear.

After names, it would be good to introduce verbs. Studies show that aphasic patients learn best if nouns such as names of objects and people was set first before verb. Though try to avoid "to be" and "to have" verbs as this comes out a bit difficult on their end. Use simple verbs as "open", "read", etc.

To find a way of relief, patients should explain their symptoms to the doctor. Together, they can determine the best treatment. Patients could already try some solutions when at home.

A start is to avoid things that can cause pain, such as hot baths, tight or easily bunched clothing, and pressure on the side of the body affected by the stroke. While sitting or lying down, support the paralyzed arm on an armrest or pillow to relieve shoulder pain from the arm's weight; the same should be done with a sling while walking. At least, patients could use heat packs or simple exercises prescribed by their physical therapist.

Many nursing home/rehab center residents still want to be useful. I ask that they help by making cat toys. pipe cleaners with bells and then wrapped around a pencil to make a coil. They loved seeing pictures of shelter cats playing with their labors of love. and great hand rehab work.

Stroke patients have a myriad of disabilities to contend with after being medically stabilized. There may be expressive and receptive language disabilities, mobility issues and with daily living activities. Stroke victims often have to relearn basic skills. An occupational therapist is a specialist who assists stroke victims with learning to cope with these difficulties.

When a stroke patient has difficulty with writing, there are writing aids to help. When trying to assist a friend or relative with relearning writing skills, always consult the occupational therapist for recommendations for writing tools.

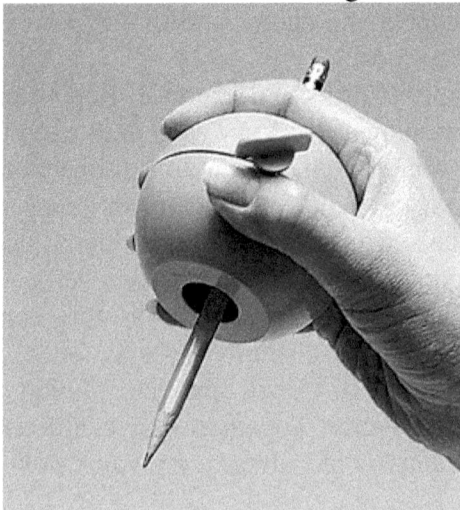

⮎ Ball is easier to grasp when finger grip is weak.

Writing Tools
Weighted Pen

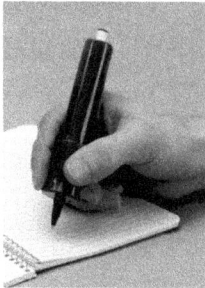

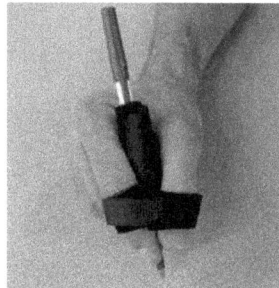

Stroke patients often have difficulty controlling writing instrument due to problems with muscle control. The Weighted Pen can help the patient grip and hold the instrument more easily. The pen comes with 8 to 10 gram weights, which can be added or removed to increase stability of the writing instrument and control writing.

Klick Pencil Holder

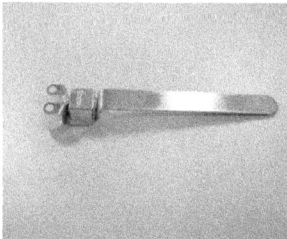

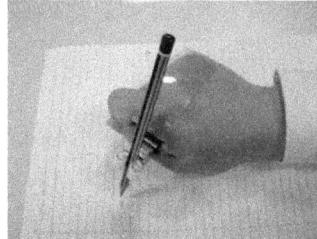

The Klick Pencil Holder is designed to hold a pencil in place so that it won't slide. It can be used with a universal cuff and by right- and left-handed individuals.

Wanchik's Writer #2

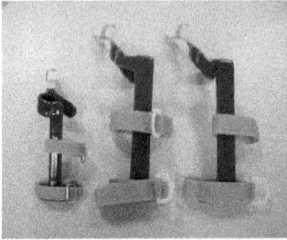

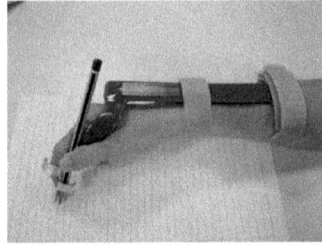

The Wanchik's Writer #2 is an orthosis which extends up the forearm, providing additional wrist support. It comes in three sizes and can be used by both children and adults. It can also be used by left- and right-handed individuals.

Slip-On Writing Aid

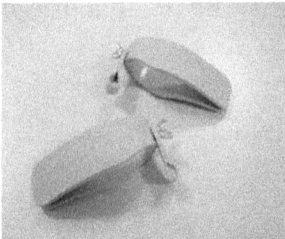

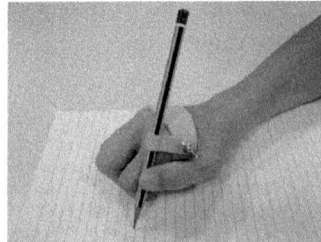

The Slip-On Writing Aid is contoured to securely fit the hand. The molded plastic writing aid holds a pen or pencil at an adjustable angle.

One-Handed Writing Board

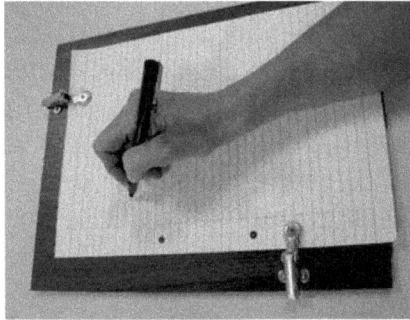

The One-Handed Writing Board has special lever-operated clamps which let the individual position the paper on the board, then lock it in place. The rubber feet under the board prevent the board from moving.

Portable Book Holder

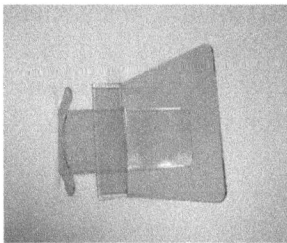

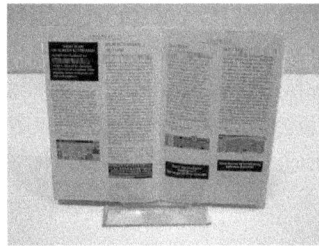

The Portable Book Holder permits hands-free reading. It is designed to allow pages to be turned easily and accommodates books of any size.

RinG-Pen Writing Instrument

This pen attachment is another option for stabilizing the writing instrument in the patient's hand. The ring fits over the index finger to help stabilize the writing instrument. Putting the finger through the ring establishes a steady grip for the stroke-disabled adult. The pen has an ergonomic design, providing a natural resting place for the finger. The pen is lightweight and provides a comfortable, steady writing instrument.

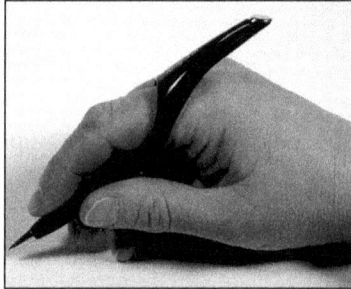

Ableware Steady Write Pen

Another choice for stabilizing the writing instrument in the patient's hand is the Steady Write Pen. This pen has a wide triangular base that increases stability. The hand balances over the triangular base as it is guided for smooth writing. Right or left handed writers can use it.

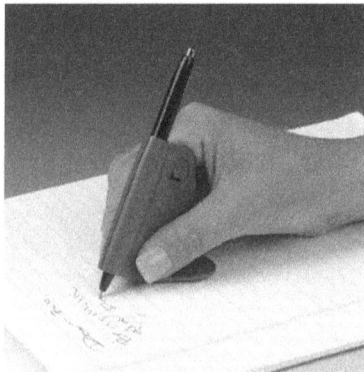

Ring Writer Clip

You can attach the Ring Writer Clip to any pen and use it with either your right or left hand. The larger ring slips over the index finger to provide stability for the writing instrument. The writing instrument slips through the smaller ring. The rings automatically position the writing instrument correctly for those who have difficulty with grip. The ring writer clip comes in three sizes to accommodate different finger sizes.

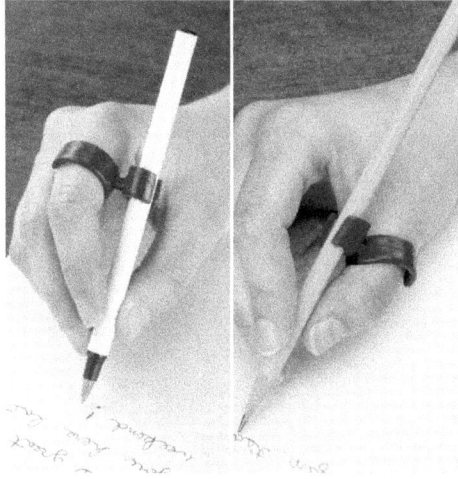

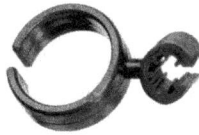

The Writing Bird

This writing instrument is another option that is beneficial to those who have difficulty holding a pen. The implement is a molded bird shaped object. The user inserts the writing instrument into a small ring at the front of the "bird." Either the right or left hand grips the bird. When you apply pressure to the tail, the pen glides smoothly over the paper.

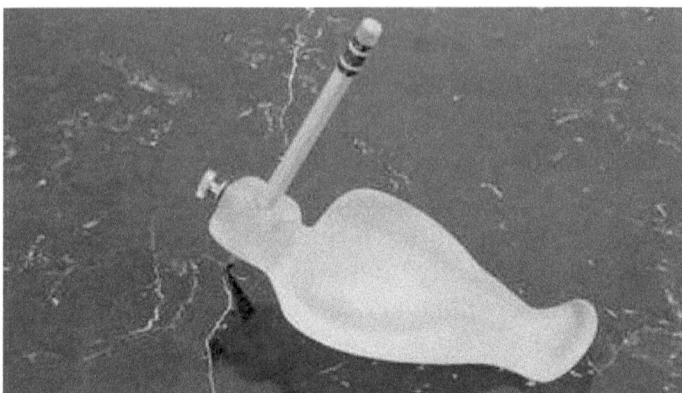

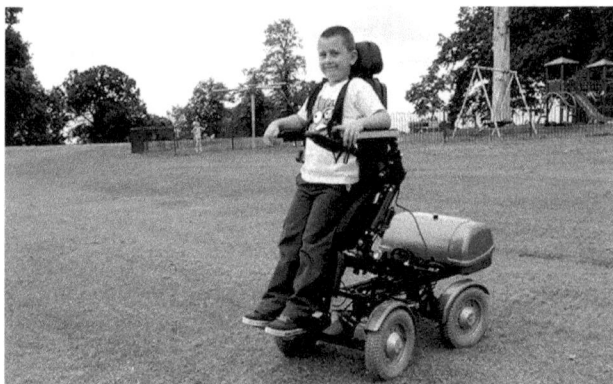

↳Boy Stands up in the Mybility All-terrain wheelchair.

Aids For Keyboard Use

Wanchik's Typer Orthoses

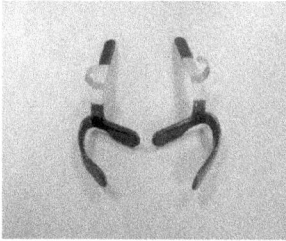

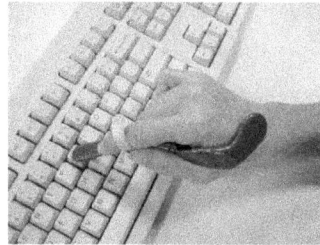

The Wanchik's Typer Orthosis permits individuals with limited hand function to type by aligning the hand in a proper and comfortable position with a palmer cuff. The rubber tip prevents the orthosis from slipping off keys. There are two sizes available for use by adults. The Wanchik's Writer #3 can be used by left- and right-handed individuals.

Slip-On Typing/Keyboard Aid

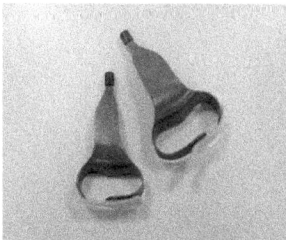

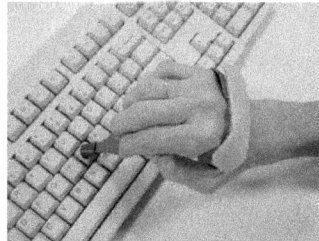

The Slip-On Typing / Keyboard Aid is designed for individuals with limited grasp. The rubber tip prevents the aid from slipping off keys. There are two sizes available and can be used by left- and right-handed individuals.

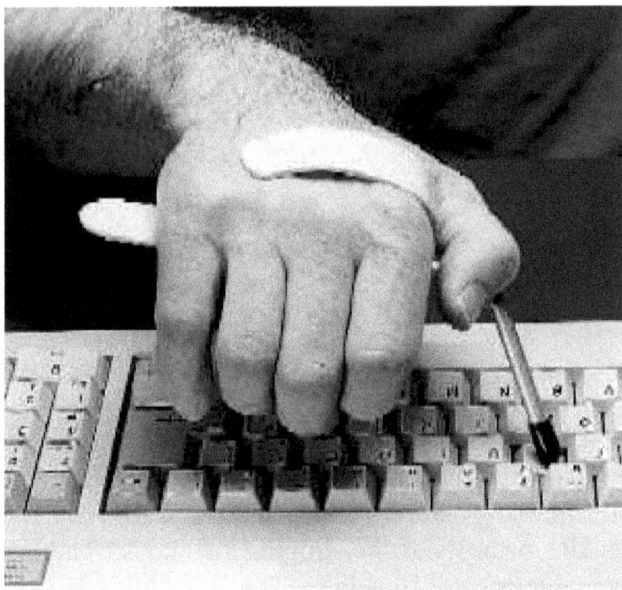

Two additional styles of keyboard assists.

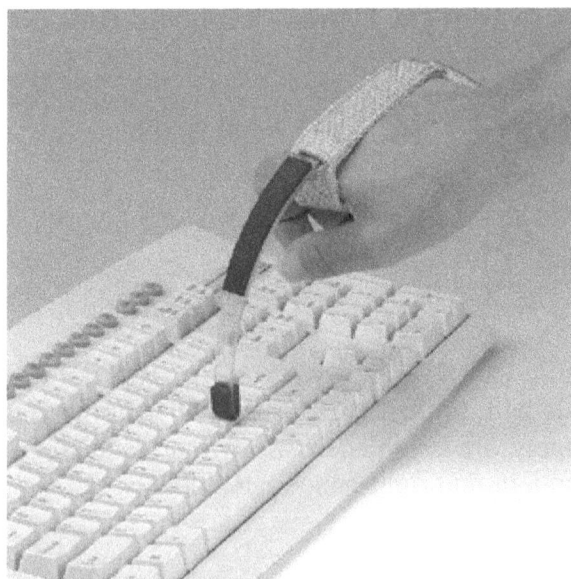

How to Stimulate Language After a Stroke

Talk about things that you enjoy – family, friends, hobbies - go through family photo albums.

Use any visuals that may be of assistance.

Try singing, or even begin by humming some of your favorite songs together! Even simple ones such as "happy birthday". Research has shown that music that is mostly stored in the right side of the brain, stimulates the damaged left side of the brain after a stroke.

Talk about things that are important – feelings, responsibilities, problems, finances.

Watch game shows that use language or math – for example, Jeopardy, Who Wants To Be A Millionaire, Family Feud, The Price Is Right, Wheel of Fortune.

Play board games that stimulate language – for example Cranium, Pictionary, Mystery Garden Game, Brain Quest, Apples to Apples, Trigon, Go to the Head of the Class, Trivia, Scattergories, Scrabble. If a game is too hard, use the easier questions, take away the timer, or buy the Junior version. Play for fun, not for points!

MOST IMPORTANTLY - You may continue doing the hobbies and activities you've always done!

Don't hesitate to search the internet for companies who specialize in handicap accessories. You might get an idea from one but find the product cheaper at another. And beware of scammers when shopping online from little-known companies.

Tips to Increase Talking After Stroke

- Allow extra time to talk.
- Noise can make it harder to listen so turn off the TV, radio, CD player.
- Sit away from the air conditioner, washing machine, dish washer.
- Don't try to talk in the car or on the street.
- Use photos or simple drawings
- Write down "key words', the most important ideas in the discussion.
- Check to see if the other person understood. If they don't understand, try to say it another way. Be flexible.
- Remember that it can be frustrating for everyone. Try to stay calm, and keep your sense of humor!

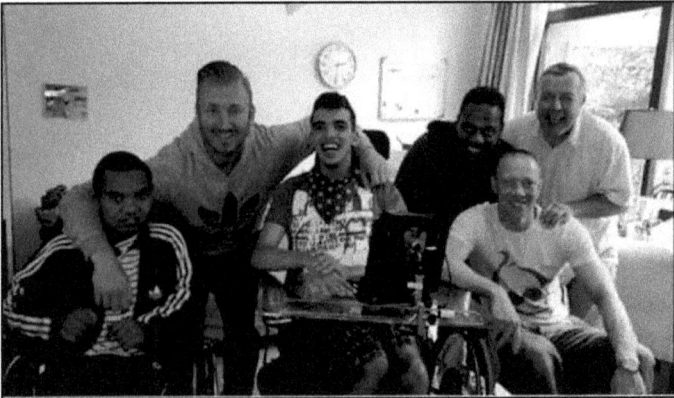

Therapy and recovery is easier when surrounded by friends.

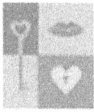

**How To Communicate
With Someone You Love:
Your Keys To Success**

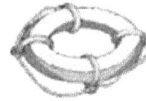

	Take time to communicate.
	Speak at a slow, normal rate.
	Talk in a quiet place.
	Write key words. Use pictures and drawings.
	Act it out.
	If it's not working, try another approach.
	Make sure you are on the same page.

Communicating with the Aphasic Patient

1) Make the patient's daily schedule of activities as routine as possible. A structured day improves the patients' orientation and memory allowing them to take on greater responsibility in their rehabilitation.

2) Try to provide communication stimulation during routine patient care activities. For example, as you feed them, talk about the foods they are eating for dinner, the

classification, the way the foods they are eating are prepared.

3) Never discuss anything in the presence of the aphasic patient that you would not want them to hear. Even the patient who's comprehension is poor may attend to body language such as facial expression, which may result in the patient becoming confused or frightened.

4) Encourage the patient to participate in group activities to promote socialization and language stimulation.

5) Don't discuss the patient's business or personal matters with them when they are fatigued or become upset. Postpone it for another time.

6) Be sure you have the patient's attention before beginning any communication. Touch them on the shoulder, wait until they are looking at you and then begin.

7) For best results, the environment in which you are communicating should be quiet and calm, and as relaxed as possible for optimal communication.

8) The patient is an adult and should be continued to be treated as one. Although there may be comprehension difficulties, they are aware that they are adults, and treating them any other way is demoralizing.

9) Speak slowly, using natural pauses. Use your natural voice. Don't shout, the patient is not deaf or hard of hearing, they are aphasic.

10) Keep instructions or questions short, simple, direct, and answerable with a "yes" or "no". Use gestures or visual cues whenever possible.

11) If the patient does not understand or respond appropriately, tell them that they did not understand you, pause, and repeat, possibly rewording it.

12) If the patient is trying to tell you something and you are unable to understand, ask simple questions and use simple gestures until they indicate that you have found the subject area.

13) If all techniques fail, and you do not know what the patient is trying to tell you, admit it, saying "I'm sorry, I don't understand. Maybe we can try again later."

14) Give the aphasic time to respond, don't interrupt, or try to fill in for them.

15) Often an aphasic patient is able to say a word one moment, but not the next, or repeat it again at a later time, Don't say, "You said it yesterday, you can say it again" By giving the patient just the beginning sound of the word they are trying to say, may be helpful. Or describing similar words or what it's used for.

16) When the aphasic patient makes a mistake, try to minimize the frustration by saying, "That's hard to get out".

17) Don't correct errors. Try re-stating what you think they were trying to get out.

18) In group situations, don't talk for the aphasic patient, or don't talk as if they were not in the room.

19) Be realistic, Telling them that "Your speech will come back" will not make them feel better in the long run. Instead, be honest, "We can't tell how much speech will return. You just have to try your best."

20) Try not to show your frustration or take your frustration out on the patient.

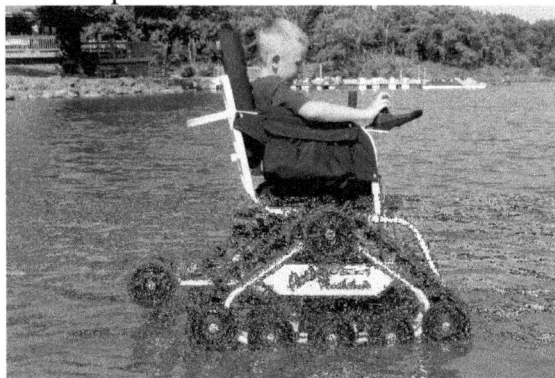

Youngster enjoying track wheelchair.

Splinting

Weakness after stroke can diminish mobility in your hand. Occupational therapists use hand-splinting techniques to reduce tightness, improve range of motion and reduce pain after stroke.

A hand splint may first be applied while you are in the hospital to reduce risk of contractures -- a condition in which fingers get "stuck" in a bent position, leading to hygiene issues and skin breakdown. Depending on your needs, splints may be pre-made or custom-molded by your therapist out of thermoplastic materials.

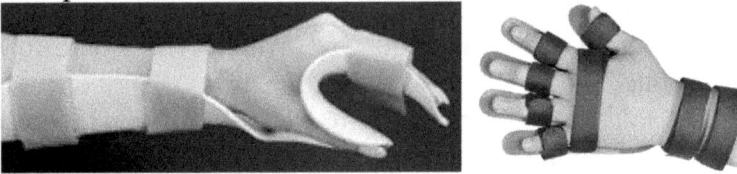

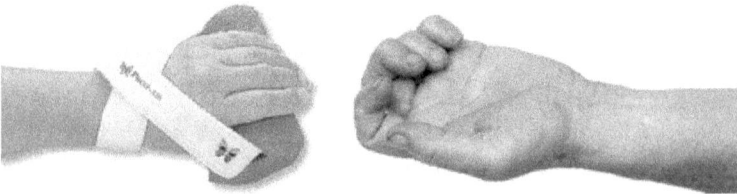

Splints may be worn temporarily until you regain use of your hand, or permanently if your hand function remains limited. Without the split, your fingers and wrist may become rigid in an distorted position.

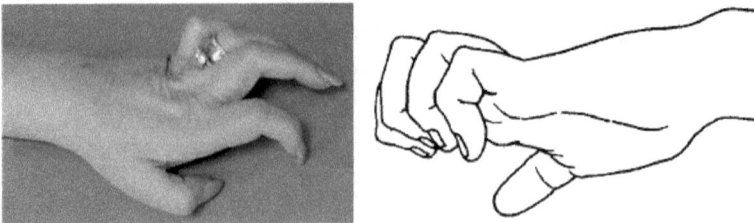

Range-of-Motion Exercises

Maintaining range of motion is one of the earliest functions of physical therapy after a stroke. Joint range of motion should be completed at a minimum daily and should involve physical or occupational therapy, nursing, the stroke survivor and any family members who are available to be trained. Range-of-motion exercises should be completed for all joints and ranges. Basic arm exercises include making a fist, waving the wrist, rotating the palm up and down, bending the elbow and raising the arm overhead.

Strengthening Exercises

Strengthening exercises are important for any muscle groups that have active muscle function, including the arm. Electrical stimulation has been used in conjunction with active muscle contractions to produce a stronger contraction and facilitate return of strength. Electrical stimulation can be used during specific tasks, such as dressing, or as an aid to strength training. Strengthening exercises for the arm include bending and straightening the elbow, lifting the arm overhead and out to the side, chair pushups and chest presses. Strengthening can be advanced by use of free weights or weightlifting equipment.

Constraint-Induced Therapy

Constraint-induced therapy may be used to promote improved arm function. Physical therapists place the unaffected arm in a sling. The person who has had a stroke then works on tasks such as dressing, writing or eating, forcing the affected arm to do all of the necessary work. In results of a randomized controlled trial published in the April 2012 issue of "Physical Therapy," participants receiving constraint-induced therapy for 2 hours per day, 5 days per week for 3 weeks had higher scores on assessments and improved quality and amount of movement compared with those who received standard rather than constraint-induced therapy.

Mental Practice

Mental practice is an area of stroke rehabilitation with a growing body of evidence. Studies have shown an improvement in performance of functional tasks when mental practice is combined with physical therapy. Mental practice or visualization of how to perform the task can aid in improved sequencing of more complex tasks as well.

For example, the task of standing up is broken into smaller steps. These might include scooting to the edge of the chair, placing the feet flat on the floor, using the hands to push up from the chair and standing up straight and tall. The stroke survivor visualizes herself doing each of these tasks separately and then in sequence to improve the quality and accuracy of movement

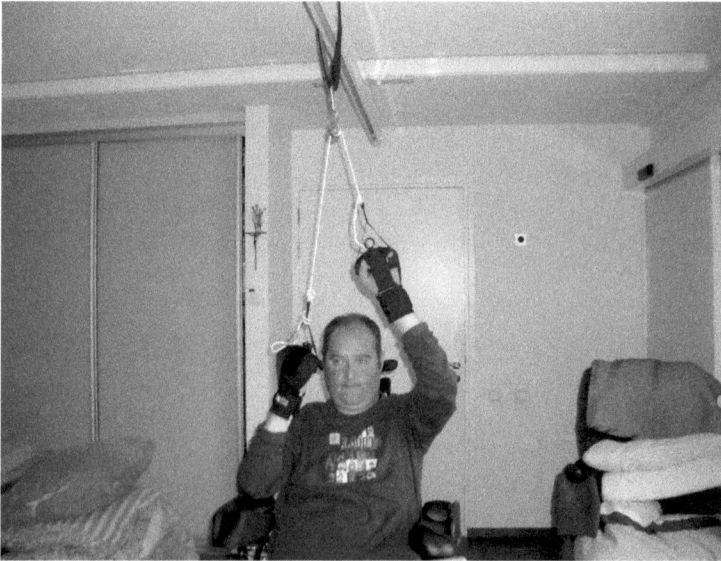

Ceiling pulley for arm exercise.

♫ Music Therapy ♫

Music therapy provided by trained music therapists may help to improve movement in stroke patients, according to a new Cochrane Systematic Review. A few small trials also suggest a wider role for music in recovery from brain injury.

More than 20 million people suffer strokes each year. Many patients acquire brain injuries that affect their movement and language abilities, which results in significant loss of quality of life. Music therapists are trained in techniques that stimulate brain functions and aim to improve outcomes for patients. One common technique is rhythmic auditory stimulation (RAS), which relies on the connections between rhythm and movement. Music of a particular tempo is used to stimulate movement in the patient.

Seven small studies, which together involved 184 people, were included in the review. Four focused specifically on stroke patients, with three of these using RAS as the treatment technique. RAS therapy improved walking speed by an average of 14 metres per minute compared to standard movement therapy, and helped patients take longer steps. In one trial, RAS also improved arm movements, as measured by elbow extension angle.

"This review shows encouraging results for the effects of music therapy in stroke patients," said lead researcher Joke Bradt of the Arts and Quality of Life Research Center at Temple University in Philadelphia, US. "As most of the studies we looked at used rhythm-based methods, we suggest that rhythm may be a primary factor in music therapy approaches to treating stroke."

Other music therapy techniques, including listening to live and recorded music, were employed to try to improve speech, behavior and pain in patients with brain injuries, and although outcomes in some cases were positive, evidence was limited. "Several trials that we identified had less than 20 participants," said Bradt. "It is expected that larger samples sizes will be used in future studies to enable sound recommendations for clinical practice."

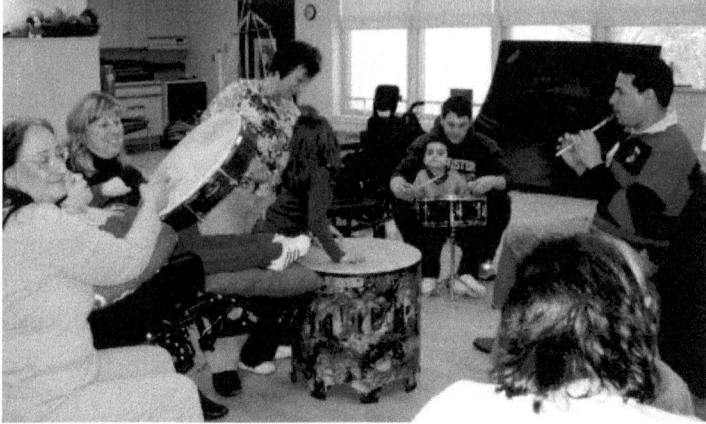

♮Three types of drums for rhythm and a recorder for melody.

What is Music Therapy?

Music Therapy is the clinical and evidence-based use of music interventions to accomplish individualized goals within a therapeutic relationship by a credentialed professional who has completed an approved music therapy program.

Music therapy interventions can be designed to:

- Promote Wellness
- Manage Stress
- Alleviate Pain
- Express Feelings
- Enhance Memory
- Improve Communication
- Promote Physical Rehabilitation

Research in music therapy supports its effectiveness in a wide variety of healthcare and educational settings.

How Music Therapy Can Help Stroke Victims

According to the American Stroke Association, music therapy has been scientifically and medically proven to be a valuable tool in rehabilitation after a stroke in areas of movement and muscle control, speech and communication, cognition, mood and motivation.

•Movement and muscle control improvement can be achieved by a steady beat, musical timing, and rhythmic patterns. Suggested activities include playing a drum to boost range of motion in the upper extremities, exercising to an upbeat music, and timing music to complement the usual walking pattern.

•To improve speech and communication in a stroke survivor, a music therapist uses rhythm, melody, and singing. Suggested activities include exercising mouth muscle, rhyming, chanting and rapping and singing the words and transferring them to speech.

•Cognition (memory, organization, attention and problem solving) can be enhanced by music. Suggested activities in this aspect include making a song with important information in its lyrics, performing in a band and rhythm repetition games.

•To enhance mood and motivation and help in pain management a music therapist uses the emotional and aesthetic qualities of music. Suggested activities in this area include listening to music, recording and song writing, improvisation and musical performance. (e.g. playing a musical instrument).

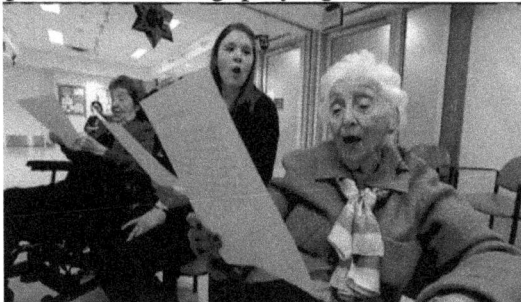

🎵Group singing improves memory and mood

The Impact of Music Therapy on Stroke Survivors

Music has been proven to have an effect on sections of the brain and an impact on social interactions and emotions. Experimental studies of music therapy have shown a significant improvement in quality of life, expression of feelings, awareness and responsiveness, positive associations, socialization and involvement with the environment.

More recent findings on music therapy suggest a decrease in depression, reduction of anxiety and improvement of mood. Researchers also suggest that music helps in motivating a positive outlook among patients. Music therapy in combination with adjunct therapies increases rehabilitation success among stroke survivors.

A Promising Study on Music Therapy and Stroke Patients

According to a Finnish researcher at the Helsinki Brain Institute, listening to music for a few hours daily can significantly improve a stroke patient's early recovery. A study on 54 patients with right or left hemisphere middle cerebral stroke showed improvement in verbal memory and focused attention after 2 months of music therapy. Patients who listened to music daily also had a more positive attitude compared to those who listened to audio books. Music should be a daily part of rehabilitation, since it is a "targeted, easy-to-conduct and inexpensive means to facilitate cognitive and emotional recovery".

The team also found that 3 months after the stroke, verbal memory improved from the first week post-stroke by 60% in music listeners. 18% in audio book listeners and 29% in non-listeners. Similarly, focused attention--the ability to control and perform mental operations and resolve conflicts among responses--improved by 17% in music listeners, but no improvement was observed in audio book listeners and non-listeners. These differences remained six months after the stroke.

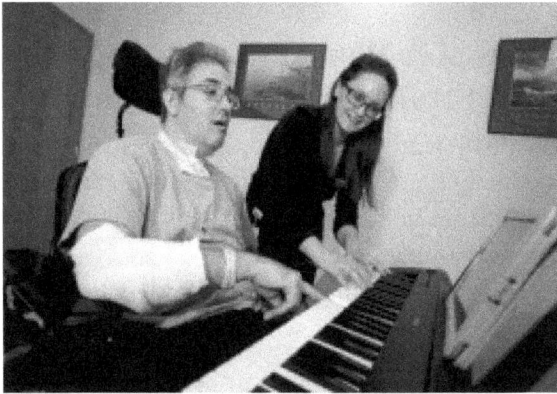

↳One-hand can play music on a keyboard.

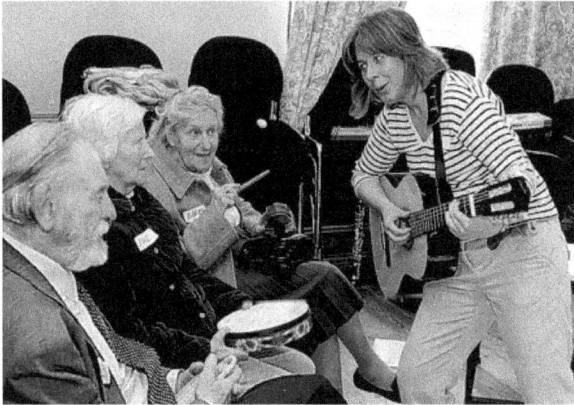

↳This group is comprised of a wooden tone block,
drum and cowbell accompanied by guitar

Story of A Woman Recovering From A Stroke Using Music Therapy

In May, 2014 Cathy was told she would never be able to move or speak again. Cathy suffered a stroke and was unable to open her mouth on her own. In less that a year she was finally able to carry on simple conversations.

"They had no clue," said her husband Billy. "They had no clue how strong she is. She's way stronger than I am".

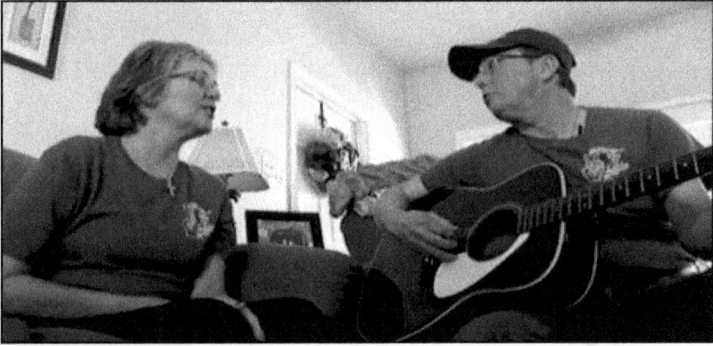

Billy said whenever his wife would yawn, therapists at the rehabilitation hospital had to place an apparatus in her mouth just to keep her mouth open to brush her teeth or to feed her food. As a musician, he naturally geared towards music therapy as an way to help his wife.

"I really think music therapy is something that bypasses the blocks that strokes cause," he said. "It gives that person a chance to communicate."

They began signing up for music therapy sessions at the hospital. The couple said though the hospital offered a limited amount of sessions, they believed music would help.

"I played music pretty much all my life," said Billy. "We were together in a band, her and three other girls and three other guys. I thought that if we had music therapy, it was just kind of something fun and good for her to do."

In a video recorded during Cathy's first music therapy session, Cathy is shown sitting down with therapists as they played Johnny Cash's "Walk The Line" when all of a sudden, Cathy begins to sing; it was the first time she opened her mouth on her own.

"I had no idea that it might lead to her being able to do what she did for the first time," he said. "I mean, I was just unbelievably touched and I was glad I had it on video. I've watched that video a thousand times."

Cathy continues to progress and can now carry on simple conversations. The couple, who dated when they were 13 and 16 and later found each other and have been married since. Billy says music has always been important to him, but he's never seen it change the quality of life in someone like it did with his wife.

"Through God's grace, she's overcome that," he said. "She doesn't even have to say anything. You can just tell."

The couple continues to attend music therapy sessions as often as they can.

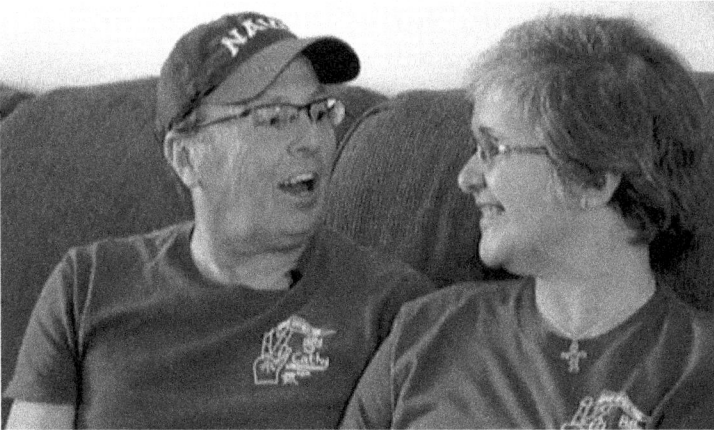

Story of Man Who Recovered
With Help From Family

My family and I live with my father. Looking at him now you might not know he's recovered from a stroke; he is an active man, walking every day and still driving. His speech and fine motor skills are good, and he can write almost as if nothing ever happened.

But it took lots of work on his part and on our part; Medicare refused to pay for professional rehabilitation help after his hospitalization. Here's how we did it together.

The months leading up to his stroke had been stressful on the whole family with the unexpected death of my mother, and my father was still emerging from his grief. It was late June, and I was getting ready for work. I noticed my father was napping, but he was in his bedroom and that was unusual.

When he woke up, my instincts told me something was wrong, so I asked him if he was feeling all right. My father shook his head and lost his balance. I looked at his face; his features were drooping. I suggested he go to the hospital. He is a proud man; he said no in a clear and resounding way--the first and only word he uttered that day.

I finally got him to the hospital after promising not to call an ambulance. Once there, we were told he had had a mild to moderate stroke. My father smokes, which raises the risk of stroke, and though the doctors don't agree, I do feel my mother's death contributed to it as well. He also had high blood pressure, which we didn't know about.

In the hospital, a wonderful team of therapists worked with him. Within a day of his returning home, several therapists evaluated him. They all said he was well enough to get by on his own, because he had some speech and could print his initials.

I soon found out that because of these recommendations Medicare would not pay for any occupational therapy--group or otherwise. It angered me that these health care workers came into my house and spent a maximum of thirty minutes with him to determine his outcome.

I tried to get him reevaluated but Medicare wouldn't budge, so I took matters into my own hands. I began researching, reading everything I could find on stroke and rehabilitation. With the help of a friend who watched and helped her father recover, I began doing what we could not pay the health providers to do. I became his therapist.

I said earlier he was a proud man and that was the first obstacle I had to overcome. I told him I knew he didn't need my help and that I was only offering it.

The second obstacle was his depression, and his feeling of being less of a person because he needed assistance doing his everyday tasks. I approached those obstacles as one, as I thought they went hand in hand.

I did small, "sneaky" things at first; I left pads of paper around his favorite places in the house with pens that were thicker. Slowly he began to pick up the pen and paper and practiced his initials. It was hard to watch his frustration, so I approached him with an idea that might help him regain the strength he needed to write.

I handed him a ball of putty. I told him to squeeze it, and twist it as if he was using his keys to open the front door. I left him alone. I came back a few minutes later and he was working with the putty. It took him about a month before he was able to write his name; though not as well as before the stroke, he was making progress.

His speech was a problem as well; it was slurred, and it took him several minutes to come up with the words he wanted to use. I really wasn't sure how to approach this, but I remembered one of the therapists left a list of exercises he could do to strengthen his facial muscles.

He felt self-conscious doing these exercises, so I suggested he do them for my then one year old daughter. I told him to make it a game and see if he could get her to mimic him. It soon became their favorite game together. My daughter found him very entertaining and my father enjoyed the laughter they shared. It wasn't long before his facial muscles were stronger.

While the muscles were gaining strength, he still had trouble with the thought process. Because he was embarrassed, he disliked talking to people. I thought of how we encourage our children to talk when they are young; why not do the same with my father? I decided to use my young daughter again.

My daughter loved to cuddle in his lap before the stroke and have him read books. I would read to her some. Then, I would whisper in her ear to take a book to Pop Pop and have him read to her. My daughter didn't care what he sounded like, she just wanted to hear the story, and the act of reading would help him practice talking without realizing it.

My young daughter willingly participated in my plan, although at a year old she did not understand the full extent of how she helped him recover. Over the next few weeks, she had him read three or four books a day. He resisted at first, but she batted her eyelashes and smiled her crooked smile, and he was doomed. The days turned into weeks, I saw his confidence grow as he read to his granddaughter. He started asking her to choose new books and began talking more freely to people outside of our household.

I helped with his bill paying for a few months, just until he had the confidence to do it by himself. One day I found him doing his bills, I asked if he wanted help. He said no; "I'll do it and have you look it over when I'm finished." I looked everything over and it was perfect. He says that was the day he regained control of his life.

Many people tell me that he couldn't have done it without me. I tell them I didn't do a thing except plant the seed of self-recovery. My father did all the hard work. He deserves all the credit for putting up with my sneaky ways of helping him recover.

Statistics and Characteristics of Stroke

Patient characteristics, including age, sex, ethnicity (white/not white), and prestroke disability (defined as a Rankin Scale score of ≤3), were collected within 48 hours of randomization. Data on the severity of stroke had been recorded within 2 weeks of the stroke and were extracted from case notes. These included the presence of urinary incontinence, dysarthria, limb deficit (weakness or paralysis in any limb), swallowing deficit, dysphasia, and level of consciousness (with the Glasgow Coma Scale), all measured at the time of maximum impairment. All stroke patients, including both ischemic and hemorrhagic stroke patients, were eligible for inclusion.

Pattern of Recovery After Stroke

The 299 subjects, 30 of whom died before the end of the study, were assessed on a total of 1346 occasions. Summary below gives result for all patients including those who were and were not assessed at every occasion.

Summary:

- Patients 80 years and up tended to improve faster than younger patients initially but then to show a sharper long-term decline.
- Patients with dysphasia tended to improve faster initially, but after approximately 12 weeks after stroke, the recovery curves for those with and without dysphasia appeared to be parallel.
- Those with no limb paralysis or weakness showed little recovery because of the "ceiling" effect of the BI.
- Those with limb deficit improved quickly initially but then showed a slightly steeper long-term decline than those with no limb deficit.

Famous People Who Survived Strokes

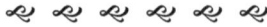

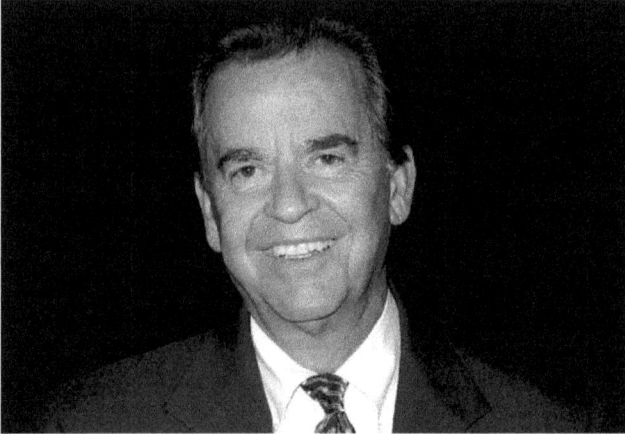

ھ ھ ھ ھ ھ ھ ھ

Dick Clark

An American television icon, Dick Clark became famous as the creator and host of "American Bandstand." He is perhaps one of the most visible celebrities to suffer a stroke. In 2004, he announced that he had type 2 diabetes, and later in the year, he was hospitalized with a stroke. This is, unfortunately, a very common complication from diabetes, and it left Clark unable to host the New Year's Eve party from Times Square that year.

He did return, but he struggled with dysarthia on his telecasts in subsequent years. However, his confidence never seemed to flag, and although he struggled to make himself clear to viewers, he continued on with his life's work of entertaining millions until his death. Following his stroke in 2004, he continued to host "Dick Clark's New Year's Rockin' Eve" and inspired millions with his strength until he died in April 2012.

ꬉ ꬉ ꬉ ꬉ ꬉ ꬉ

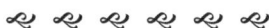

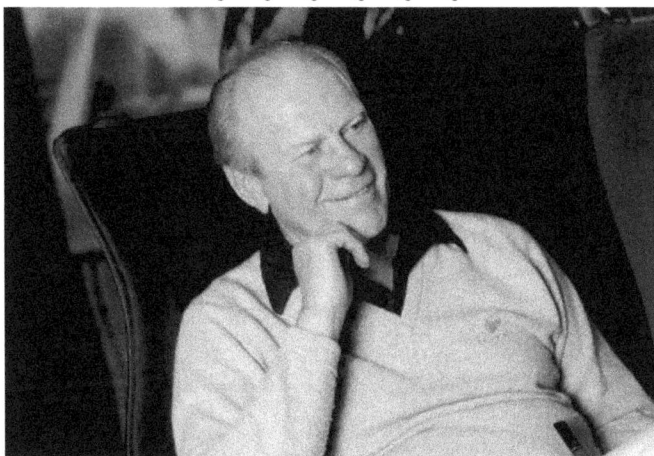

President Gerald Ford

Before becoming the 38th U.S. President, Ford was a star on the University of Michigan football team and a lieutenant commander in the Navy during WWII. He suffered a stroke during the 2000 Republican Convention at age 87. Other U.S. presidents who have experienced a stroke: Thomas Jefferson, Dwight D. Eisenhower, Franklin D. Roosevelt, Woodrow Wilson, and Ford's predecessor, Richard Nixon.

෨ ෨ ෨ ෨ ෨ ෨

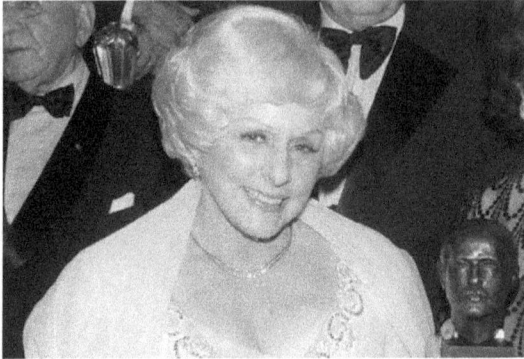

Mary Kay Ash

Mary Kay Ash started a cosmetics company in 1963 with $5,000. Today, the cosmetics giant, Mary Kay, Inc., has been named one of the best companies to work for in America by Fortune magazine. Ash suffered a stroke in 1996 that ended her career.

෨ ෨ ෨ ෨ ෨ ෨

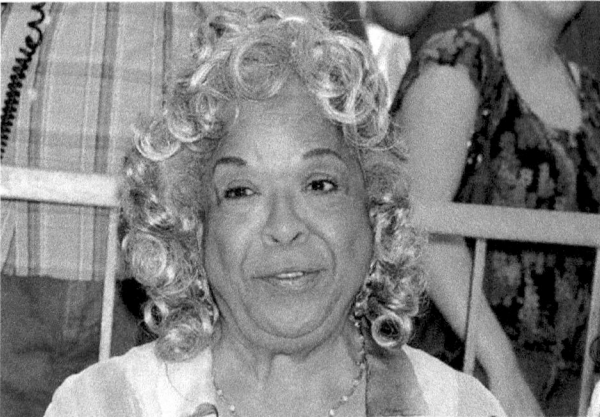

Della Reese

The former "Touched by an Angel" star survived an aneurysm during an appearance on "The Tonight Show" When a blood vessel burst in her brain, it turned into a hemorrhagic stroke. Later, she became a spokeswoman for the National Stroke Association.

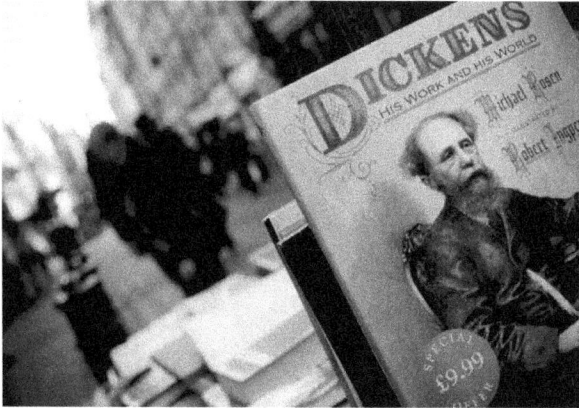
Charles Dickens

Born in 1812, Dickens was the mind behind great literary works including "Oliver Twist," "Great Expectations," and "A Tale of Two Cities." He suffered a stroke on June 8, 1870, at age 58 and died the next day.

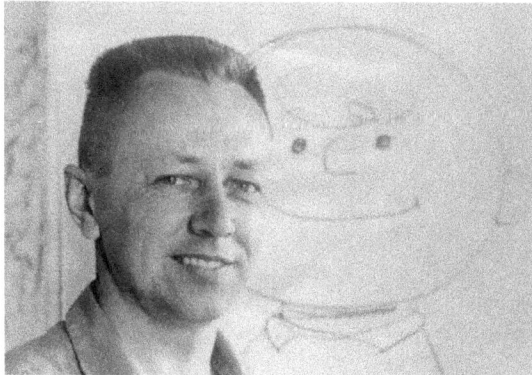
Charles Schulz

At one point, more than 150 million newspaper readers followed this cartoonist's "Peanuts" gang. In 1999, at age 77, Schulz retired after suffering a stroke and being diagnosed with colon cancer. Schulz's cartoon collections have sold more than 300 million copies in 26 languages.

ช ช ช ช ช ช

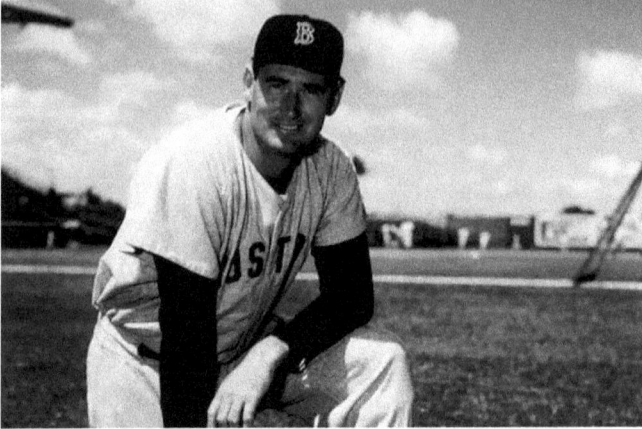

Ted Williams

The Boston Red Sox slugger had his finest year in 1941, when he hit .406. He ended his 21-year career with the team in 1960. Six years later, he was elected to the Baseball Hall of Fame. Williams suffered a stroke in 1994 and lived until 2002. He is still a Boston legend.

ช ช ช ช ช ช

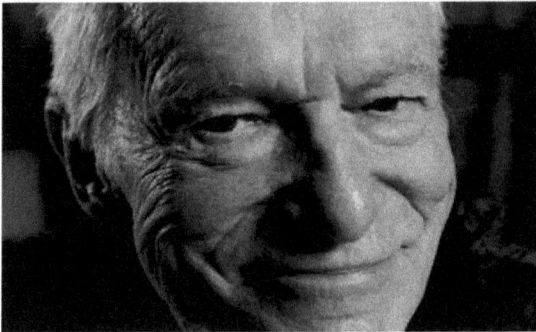

Hugh Hefner

The controversial magazine publisher who launched the Playboy media empire in his late 20s suffered a stroke in his late 50s. He later described this incident in 1985 as a "stroke of luck" for how it changed the direction of his life. A few years after the stroke, the famous bachelor married, though that marriage officially ended in 2010.

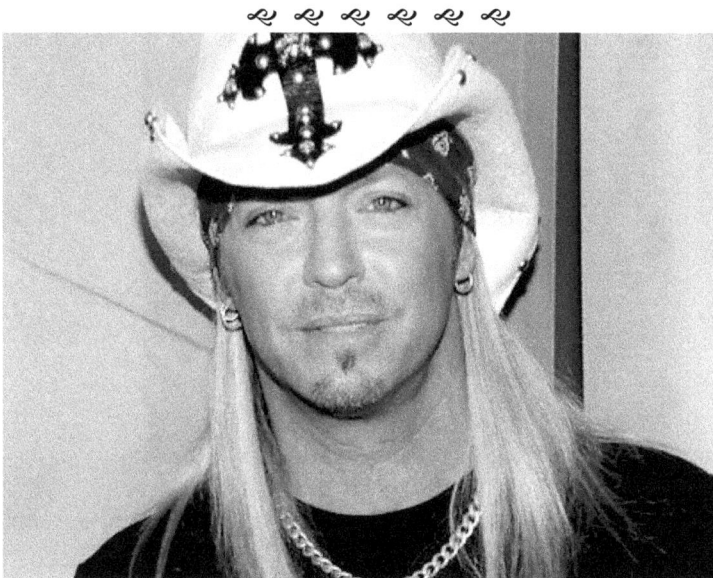

Bret Michaels

In 2010, former rocker Bret Michaels was rushed to the hospital with abdominal pain. At that time, it was found that he had appendicitis, and the offending organ was successfully removed.

However, later on in the year, he had a blinding headache and was readmitted into the hospital. He had suffered a massive subarachnoid hemorrhage, bleeding around the brain, which nearly killed him.

Later on in the year, Michaels had a transient ischemic attack that was found to be due to an underlying specific heart defect, patent foramen ovale. For the most part, he's made a complete recovery. Michaels is only 49 years old, and he has bounced back to continue performing and pursuing his life's goals.

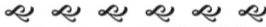

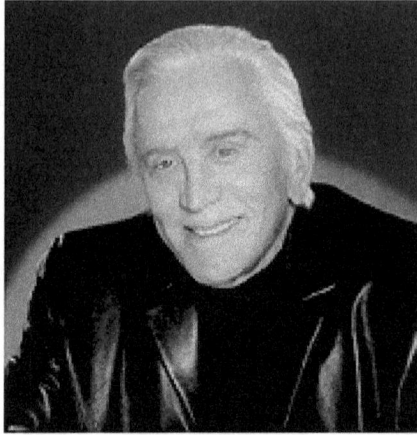

ల్ ల్ ల్ ల్ ల్ ల్

Kirk Douglas

Kirk Douglas is a handsome star of the stage and screen. He is well known for the movies in his youth and his famous son, but some know him as an example of what life is like after a stroke. In 1996, he had a stroke that permanently affected his ability to speak clearly. Working tirelessly with speech therapists, he was able to make a moving acceptance speech when awarded an honorary Academy Award in the same year.

He is still going strong at 95 years old, and he is currently the oldest active celebrity blogger. Although the stroke may have affected his ability to speak, it did not keep him from communicating through new media with the world at large.

Most people dread the thought of major life changes being thrust upon them. And fewer still would credit an unexpected health challenge as a bit of good fortune.

But actor Kirk Douglas reports that the stroke he suffered in 1996 changed him in ways that enriched his life, and ultimately became the subject of his recent book, *My Stroke of Luck*.

"You know, stroke is a very interesting thing, although at times I wish I didn't have it," says Douglas. "It makes you appreciate things. For instance, the 'simple' miracle of speech — we have no cognizance of the many intricate movements it takes to communicate verbally until it is taken away from us."

Douglas didn't consider his fate to be improved during his initial struggles with recovery. Among other problems, he had to contend with the reality that, initially, he could not talk.

"What is an actor who can't speak — do you wait for silent movies to come back?" jokes Douglas. But the Hollywood great found that even this difficult challenge was a small part in an overall struggle to reclaim his life.

Douglas soon found himself in the throes of depression. At his lowest point, he loaded the pistol he'd used in Gunfight at the OK Corral, and placed it inside his mouth.

"I know it's melodramatic," says Douglas. "But it didn't seem so at the time. Depression had me by the throat."

He was able to regain perspective at the last moment when the metallic barrel of the gun bumped against his sensitive teeth. "It hurt, and soon I found myself laughing hysterically, because I suddenly felt I was playing a part in a movie," says Douglas.

Douglas ultimately vanquished his depression with a personal epiphany.

"I found that when I began to think about the well-being of other people… I began to feel better," says Douglas. "What ultimately got me out of bed? Of course my wife and my family's support were essential, but the most important factor was the realization that I was thinking too much about my own misfortune."

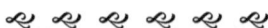

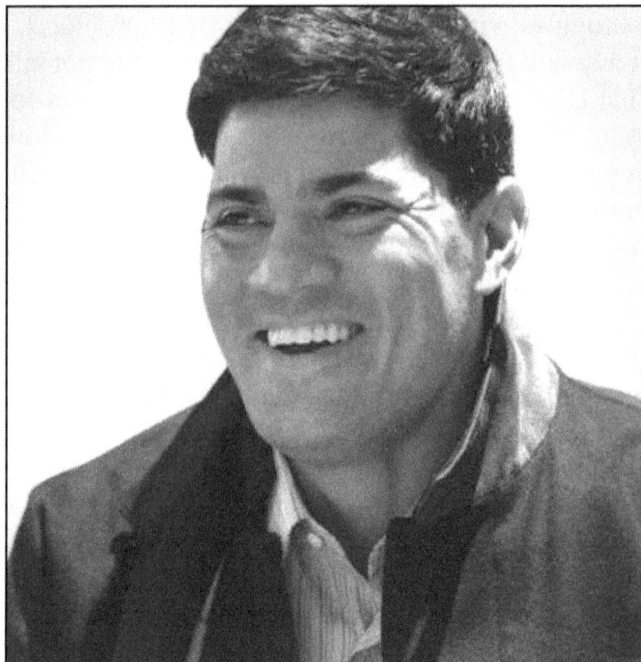

ॐ ॐ ॐ ॐ ॐ ॐ

Tedy Bruschi

At age 31—just weeks after winning his third Super Bowl—New England Patriots linebacker Tedy Bruschi suffered a debilitating stroke. He had just finished playing in a pro bowl in 2005 when he started to have numbness, blurry vision, and a headache. It was found that he had a mild stroke that was caused by a congenital hole in his heart.

Although he did experience one sided paralysis, Bruschi was cleared to play again within a year. He was elected a defensive team captain and went on to several more years of football. He retired in 2009 and currently heads up a foundation to raise stroke awareness.

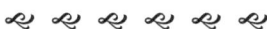

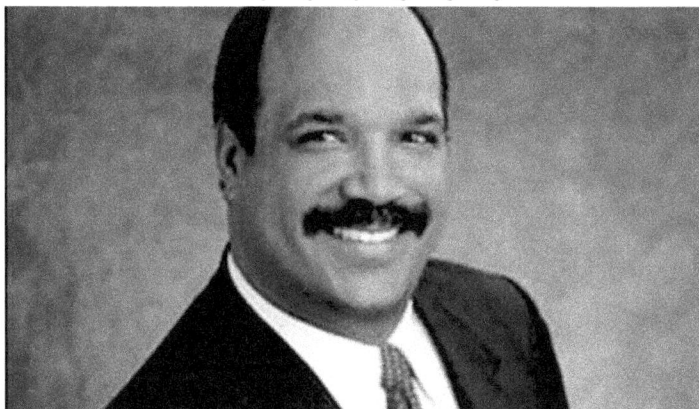

∾ ∾ ∾ ∾ ∾ ∾

Mark McEwen

Mark McEwen began his professional career as a weatherman, but he eventually parlayed that on camera work into being a features reporter for the popular CBS This Morning show. He had interviewed famous politicians and celebrities alike, but in 2005, he came up against the toughest struggle of his life. He had a massive stroke and fought for his life for several days.

When he finally recovered, he had one-sided paralysis and was confined to a wheelchair. He didn't let that stop him, though. He worked with physical therapists to eventually move to a walker and then to walk on his own.

Even though the stroke did partially affect his ability to speak, McEwen was able to rehabilitate his speaking voice and return to broadcasting in 2012. He wrote a book detailing his journey back entitled *"Change in the Weather: Life after Stroke"*. He is still anchoring the news for a California CBS affiliate.

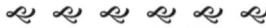

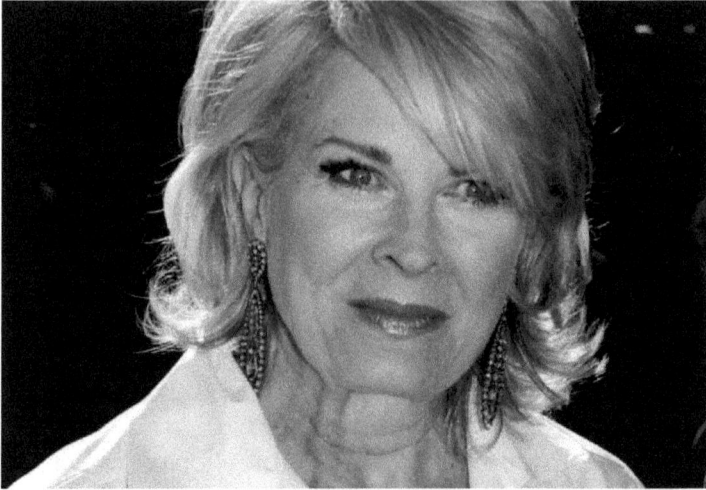

Candice Bergen

Candice Bergen is known for her supermodel looks and her Emmy award winning work on the Murphy Brown Show. It is not well known, but she also suffered a stroke in 2006. She really did not want to talk about it because she was afraid people in Hollywood would discriminate against her. So, she kept it to herself and kept moving on.

Only now is she talking about what she went through, and she admits that her memory is not what it used to be. It is the only sign she has of the stroke, but she has not let it stop her. She agreed to be in a stage play recently, and she finds it is helping her cope with her stroke – even if it takes her a bit longer to learn her lines.

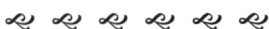

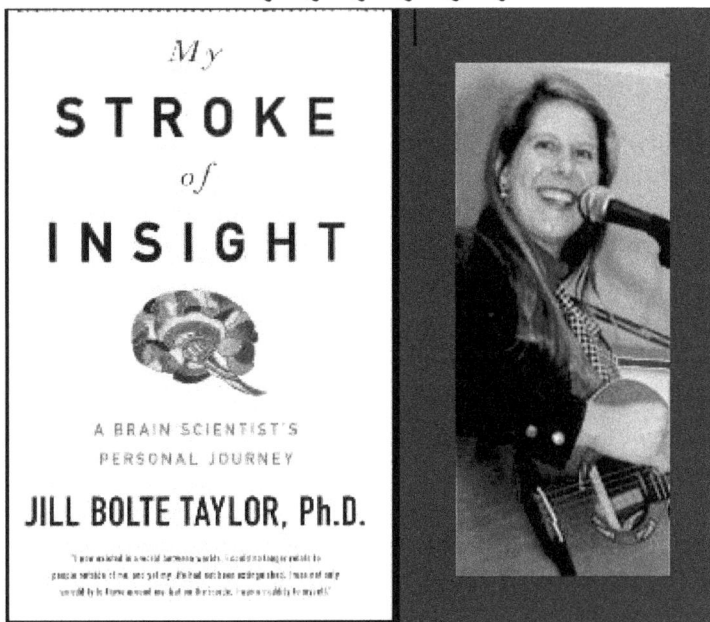

Jill Bolte Taylor

Jill Bolte Taylor was a 37-year-old Harvard-trained and published brain scientist when a blood vessel exploded in her brain. Through the eyes of a curious neuroanatomist, she watched her mind completely deteriorate whereby she could not walk, talk, read, write, or recall any of her life.

Because of her understanding of how the brain works, her respect for the cells composing her human form, and an amazing mother, Jill completely recovered her mind, brain and body.

In *My Stroke of Insight: A Brain Scientist's Personal Journey*, Jill shares with us her recommendations for recovery and the insight she gained into the unique functions of the right and left hemispheres of her brain. Having lost the categorizing, organizing, describing, judging and critically analyzing skills of her left brain, along with its language centers and thus ego center, Jill's consciousness shifted away from normal reality.

In the absence of her left brain's neural circuitry, her consciousness shifted into present moment thinking whereby she experienced herself "at one with the universe."

Based upon her academic training and personal experience, Jill helps others not only rebuild their brains from trauma, but helps those of us with normal brains better understand how we can 'tend the garden of our minds' to maximize our quality of life. Jill pushes the envelope in our understanding about how we can consciously influence the neural circuitry underlying what we think, how we feel, and how we react to life's circumstances. Jill teaches us through her own example how we might more readily exercise our right hemispheric circuitry with the intention of helping all human beings become more humane.

"I believe the more time we spend running the deep inner peace circuitry of our right brain, then the more peace we will project into the world, and ultimately the more peace we will have on the planet."

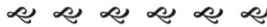

જ જ જ જ જ જ
Happy Birthday Stephen Hawking
January 8, 2015

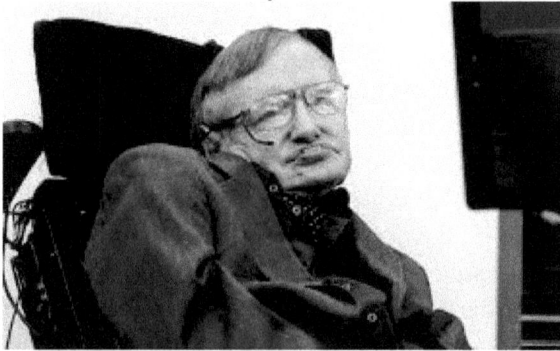

Stephen Hawking turned 73 on January 8, 2015, defeating the odds of a daunting diagnosis by over half a century. The famous theoretical physicist popularized modern cosmology, brought theories and facts about black holes and quantum gravity to the main stream and ultimately to the silver screen. The success of his works and the power his name resounds demonstrates just how massive an impact this man has had, and no doubt will continue to have on the world and its inhabitants.

A brief history of Stephen Hawking:

1942 – Born in Oxford, England, on January 8th, the 200th anniversary of the death of astronomer and physicist Galileo Galilei.

1950 – Attended St. Albans High School for Girls, but only for a few months because at the time younger boys could attend one of the houses.

1958 – Attended college at Oxford where his passion was math and his degree was in natural sciences.

1958 – While at Oxford, he coxed a rowing team, as he put it, "To relieve immense boredom".

1962 – Graduated from Oxford and went to Cambridge for his PhD.

1963 – Is diagnosed with a motor neuron disease, amyotrophic lateral sclerosis (ALS), and given the prognosis of two to three years to live.

1965 – Married first wife Jane "Wilde" Hawking.

1966 – Completed his doctoral work in theoretical physics, after submitting a thesis on black holes.

1979 – Had third child with wife Jane by the time he was 27 (showing that in addition to his brain, another body part still worked perfectly well).

1970 – Discovery of the fact that black holes emit radiation (result of combining the theory of relativity with quantum theory).

1979 – Became the 17th Lucasian Professor of Mathematics, an academic chair at Cambridge University, the same position held by Sir Isaac Newton from 1669 to 1702.

1982 – Awarded the honor of Commander of the Order of the British Empire (CBE).

1985 – Hospitalized with pneumonia and receives an emergency tracheotomy, causing permanent damage to the larynx and vocal cords. As such a keyboard operated electronic speech synthesizer is made and adapted to his wheelchair, engineered by David Mason, at the time married to Elaine Mason, one of Hawking's nurses and future second wife.

1988 – A Brief History of Time: From the Big Bang to Black Holes is published on April Fool's Day. It has become a landmark volume in scientific writing with more than 9 million copies in 40 languages sold worldwide. It remained a London Times' best-seller for more than four years.

1991 – Steven Spielberg produced Errol Morris's documentary A Brief History of Time documenting Hawking's life and accomplishments, which became so successful that it led to the publication of a reader's companion to the film and book. The success of the companion the led to a six-part television miniseries, Stephen Hawkin's Universe, first televised in 1997.

1995 – Divorced Jane married Elaine Mason (whom he divorces in 2006).

1996 – Published The Illustrated A Brief History of Time.

2004 – Reversed the 1966 theory that black holes swallow everything in their path forever and declares that black holes will never support space travel to other universes.

2007 – At 65 years old, experienced space simulation at Kennedy Space Center where he reacted.

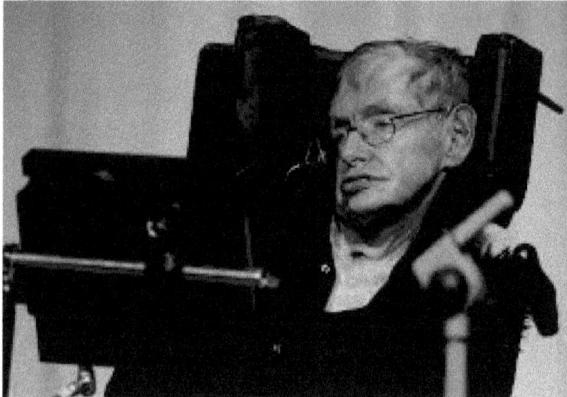

Technical Description of Stroke Afflictions

Pulmonary (lung) Aspiration

Difficulty swallowing (dysphagia) means it takes more time and effort to move food or liquid from your mouth to your stomach. Dysphagia may also be associated with pain. In some cases, swallowing may be impossible.

Pulmonary (lung) aspiration is the entry of material (such as pharyngeal secretions, food or drink, or stomach contents) from the oropharynx or gastrointestinal tract into the larynx (voice box) and lower respiratory tract (from the trachea—i.e., windpipe—to the lungs). A person may either inhale the material, or it may be delivered into the tracheobronchial tree during positive pressure ventilation. When pulmonary aspiration occurs during eating and drinking, the aspirated material is often colloquially referred to as "going down the wrong pipe."

Aspiration occurs whenever food enters the airway below the true vocal folds. Aspiration can occur before, during, or after the swallow.

Aspiration before the swallow

Aspiration occurs before the swallow in the case of a delayed or absent initiation of the swallow. It may also be the result of poor tongue control, which allows food to trickle into the pharynx while the patient is still chewing. Apparently, a "neurological override" exists which prevents the initiation of the swallow while one is still chewing

Aspiration during the swallow

Aspiration occurs during the swallow when the vocal folds fail to adduct or the larynx fails to elevate. (Remember that this type of dysphagia is uncommon. Only 5% of dysphagias involve problems with airway closure).

Aspiration after the swallow

Aspiration can occur after the swallow in several different circumstances.The patient may pocket food in the oral cavity.

Later, when he or she lies down to sleep, the food will fall down into the airway.

Food may get stuck in the pharyngeal recesses. This happens to everyone, but someone with a normal system would realize that the food was there and swallow again. A CVA or TBI patient may have a sensory impairment and allow the food to drop into the larynx.

Due to reduced laryngeal elevation, food may remain on top of the larynx.

Technical Analysis of Dysphagia

The most common type of dysphagia is delayed or absent initiation of the pharyngeal stage of the swallow. Eighty percent of CVA patients who have dysphagia have this type of problem.

It is common for patients with this type of disorder to keep trying to push the bolus into the pharynx with the tongue. Eventually, they will succeed. Where the food goes when this happens depends on three things: the posture of the patient, the consistency of the food and size of the bolus. Smaller amounts of thick substances will generally lodge in the pharyngeal recesses rather than going directly down the airway.

As a patient moves the tongue and tries to push the bolus into the pharynx, the movements of the tongue and the hyoid bone look a lot like a swallow. It will be difficult to tell whether or not the patient is aspirating. A number of patients aspirate without coughing. Also, food may be lodging in the pharyngeal recesses, which will hold several teaspoons of material, before being aspirated.

Disorders of the pharyngeal stage of the swallow are the most prevalent type of dysphagia among the CVA population; over 90% have pharyngeal stage problems. Reduced tongue driving force or poor pharyngeal stripping action is an especially common problem among those who have had CVAs. This causes food residue to accumulate in the valleculae and may lead to aspiration after the swallow. Pharyngeal stripping action is usually the last part of the swallowing process to recover. No specific site of lesion is associated with this problem.

The majority of patients who are NPO (nothing by mouth) have pharyngeal stage problems.

Fifty percent of those who have pharyngeal stage problems also have oral stage problems.

Half of CVA patients with dysphagia have problems that affect the oral stage of the swallow. Fifty percent of those have reduced or abnormal tongue movements that affect the initiation of the swallow. Typically, tongue control problems are not sufficiently severe to cause aspiration. No specific site of lesion is associated with tongue movement problems.

Only 5% of CVA patients have problems with vocal fold adduction. This type of difficulty only occurs with brain stem (cranial nerve x) lesions.

There are generally no problems with airway closure following a cortical stroke, unless there are bi-lateral upper motor neuron lesions (pseudo bulbar palsy).

Only 5% of CVA patients have swallowing problems caused by the failure of the cricopharyngeus muscle (p.e. segment) to relax. If the p.e. segment does fail to relax, food will build up in the pharynx and may be aspirated. In this case food residue will be accumulated in the pyriform sinuses, or in cases of severe problems, throughout the lower portion of the pharynx, and may cause aspiration after the swallow.

Typically, each patient will have more than one type of swallowing problem.

Site of Lesion and Related Swallowing Problems

There is currently enough evidence to specify the specific type of swallowing problem associated with particular sites of lesion caused by stroke.

Brain stem stroke typically causes the most severe cases of dysphagia. Damage to the medulla is particularly devastating as is to be expected since the "swallowing center" and the nuclei of most of the cranial nerves involved in swallowing are located there. As the cranial nerves are lower motor neurons, they form the final common pathway for all motor (pyramidal and extrapyramidal tracts) impulses traveling from the brain to the muscles involved in deglutition and speech.

Many people with brainstem strokes cannot eat and drink safely due to the risk of aspiration." Patients with unilateral medullary lesions may have functional or even normal oral control. However, they usually have significant problems with the pharyngeal stage of the swallow (the cranial nerves that innervate the pharynx and larynx originate in the medulla).

They may have one or more of the following problems: extreme delay in the initiation of the swallow response (10-15 seconds) and reduction in both elevation and anterior movement of the larynx. This in turn may lead to reduced opening of the criopharyngeus muscle. They may also have unilateral pharyngeal weakness and unilateral vocal fold paralysis. In some cases, patients will not recover their swallow for 4 to 6 months if ever.

Subcortical stroke can affect both sensory and motor pathways. It may cause problems in both the oral and pharyngeal stages of the swallow, including:

- Mild delays in oral transit time (3-5 seconds)
- Mild delays in initiation of the pharyngeal swallow (2-3 seconds)
- Impairments in the timing of the neuromuscular components of the pharyngeal swallow.

Unilateral Left Hemisphere Stroke (Cortical)

A lesion in this area may cause apraxia of the swallow. The tongue may not respond to food or may make searching movements prior to transporting the bolus. Patients with this kind of problem may have more success with oral feeding if they are allowed to feed themselves. This makes the swallow more "automatic." Other problems that occur with this type of lesion include:

- Mild delays in oral transit (3-5 seconds)
- Mild delays in the initiation of the pharyngeal swallow (2-3 seconds)
- The pharyngeal stage should be normal once it is initiated since it does not require a lot of cortical input.
- Unilateral Right Hemisphere Stroke (Cortical)
- The following problems may be experienced:
- Mild oral transit delays (2-3 seconds)
- Slightly longer pharyngeal delays (3-5 seconds)

Delayed Laryngeal Elevation

The dysphagias produced by right hemisphere lesions while anatomically and physiologically no more severe than those resulting from left hemisphere damage have poorer outcomes. Patients with right hemisphere damage tend to have attentional problems and exhibit poor judgment including impulsivity. These characteristics reduce their ability to use compensatory strategies for safe swallowing.

Multiple Strokes often cause significant swallowing problems that affect both the oral and the pharyngeal stages. Also, cognitive ability may be impaired, reducing the patient's ability to use compensatory strategies. According to Logemann (1989), the swallow is never quite the same after a stroke even when a patient is able to return to a regular diet. When a patient has another stroke later, the already compromised mechanism is further damaged.

In recovery of the swallow, tongue movement is generally the first part of the process to improve, followed by the initiation of the swallow. Pharyngeal stripping action is usually the last part of the process to improve in recovery.

Recovery is most rapid in the first 3 or 4 weeks after a stroke. Therefore, an SLP should always re-evaluate an NPO patient about one month after a stroke.

Generally, if the swallow is going to recover it will do so within 6 or 7 weeks after a stroke.

Aphasia • Speech and Language After CVA

Aphasia is a combination of a speech and language disorder caused by damage to the brain. Most often caused by a cerebral vascular accident, also known as a stroke, aphasia can cause impairments in speech and language. To be diagnosed with aphasia, a person's speech or language must be significantly impaired in one (or several) of the four communication modalities following acquired brain injury or have significant decline over a short time period (progressive aphasia).

The four communication modalities are auditory comprehension, verbal expression, reading and writing, and functional communication. The difficulties of people with aphasia can range from occasional trouble finding words to losing the ability to speak, read, or write, **but does not affect intelligence**.

This also affects visual language such as sign language. In contrast, the use of formulaic (standard pattern) expressions in everyday communication is often preserved. One prevalent deficit in the aphasias is anomia, which is a deficit in word finding ability. The term "aphasia" implies that one or more communication modalities are functioning incorrectly. Aphasia is not usually used when the language problem is a result of a more peripheral motor or sensory difficulty, such as paralysis affecting the speech muscles or a general hearing impairment.

Who May Authorize Hospice and Who's eligible?

If you have Medicare Part A (Hospital Insurance) AND meet all of these conditions, you can get hospice care:

- Your hospice doctor and your regular doctor (if you have one) certify that you're terminally ill (with a life expectancy of 6 months or less).
- You accept palliative care (for comfort) instead of care to cure your illness.
- You sign a statement choosing hospice care instead of other Medicare-covered treatments for your terminal illness and related conditions.

Only your hospice doctor and your regular doctor (if you have one) - not a nurse practitioner that you've chosen to serve as your attending medical professional - can certify that you're terminally ill and have a life expectancy of 6 months or less.

Care For Your Other Conditions

Your hospice benefit covers your care and you shouldn't have to go outside of hospice to get care (except in very rare situations). Once you choose hospice care, your hospice benefit should cover everything you need.

You must pay the deductible and coinsurance amounts for all Medicare-covered services to treat health problems that aren't part of your terminal illness and related conditions. You also must continue to pay Medicare premiums, if necessary.

What a Speech Pathologist Does
for a Stroke Victim

Speech Pathologist Job Description: Under limited supervision, provides services to identify, remedial, rehabilitate and educate individuals who have **cognitive, communication and/or swallowing disorders**. Encompasses evaluation, treatment and consultation with the goal being to maximize functional independence. Provides direct or indirect patient care and educational programs to contracting agencies. Adheres to the principles of Service Care

Miniminum Qualifications:

1) Graduate of a Speech/Language Pathology program from an accredited ASHA PSB school. Master's Degree required. Must pass ASHA certification examination and be eligible for CFY or hold CCC-SLP.
2) Must have current licensure as a Speech/Language Pathologist by the State of Iowa.
3) Typically entry level for applicants with zero to five years of recent clinical experience.
4) BCLS certification required.
5) Must be able to demonstrate achievement of Staff Speech Pathologist duties and responsibilities within the first six months of employment.
6) Is able to communicate effectively with all members of the health care team.
7) Is able to perform a variety of duties characterized by frequent change.
8) Demonstrates ability to assess and treat patients for speech pathology.

What does a speech-language pathologist (SLP) do
when working with individuals after a stroke?

As part of a medical team, the SLP diagnoses and treats cognitive-communication and swallowing deficits after a stroke. The treatment program focuses on improving the skills that have been affected by the stroke, depending on what areas are affected.

To improve the patient's ability to understand or produce language, the SLP will work on specific drills and strategies, such as:

- retraining word retrieval;
- having the patient participate in group therapy sessions to practice conversational skills with other stroke survivors;
- holding structured discussions, focusing on improving initiation of conversation, turn-taking, clarification of ideas, and repairing of conversational breakdowns;
- role-playing common communication situations that take place in the community and at home, such as talking on the telephone or ordering a meal in a restaurant.

Later in the recovery process, the SLP may work with a vocational specialist to help transition the person back into work or school, if applicable. The SLP may also work with the employer and/or an educational specialist to implement the use of compensatory strategies—for example, modifying the patient's work/school environment to meet language and/or cognitive needs.

Individuals may also require speech-language pathology services to improve speech production if they have difficulty due to muscle weakness or deficits in motor programming. They may also be taught strategies to make speech more intelligible and to compensate for the muscle weakness. The SLP can also evaluate a person's ability to use augmentative or alternative communication (AAC) devices and techniques to supplement the individual's verbal communication.

The SLP can evaluate a person's swallowing function and make recommendations that involve positioning issues, feeding techniques, diet consistency changes, and education of the person with stroke, family members, or caregivers.

If cognitive skills are affected, some treatment strategies may include:

using a memory log to keep track of daily happenings to help with memory;

using an organizer to plan tasks;

increasing awareness of deficits in order to help self-monitoring in the hospital, home, and community.

How Effective Are Treatments For A Stroke?

ASHA has written a treatment efficacy summary for cognitive-communication disorders resulting from right hemisphere brain damage that describes evidence about how well treatment works. This summary is useful not only to individuals with stroke and their caregivers, but also to insurance companies considering payment for much-needed services for stroke.

Specifically for adults with RHD (Right Hemisphere Brain damage), data from ASHA's National Outcomes Measurement System (NOMS) show that for patients with right hemisphere cerebrovascular disease who received speech- language pathology services:

- 73% improved in problem solving
- 80% increased attention
- 74% improved memory
- 77% improved in pragmatics.

Treatments for visuospatial neglect have been shown to be effective primarily when they are intensive, encourage active scanning or internal cueing (as opposed to clinician-driven cues, such as "look to the left"), or involve left limb movement combined with scanning tasks. For broader cognitive-communication abilities, one outcome study of individuals with RHD evaluated the benefits of a program that focused on physical, emotional, vocational, speech and language function along with family education and support. Although improvement was not seen in all deficit areas, results suggested that the participants developed greater independence in daily living and returned to modified work programs.

Speech-Language Pathologist Continued

The role of the Speech-Language Pathologist is to assess patients   with RHD to identify the specific deficits that are present along with preserved abilities and areas   of relative strength in order to   maximize functional independence   and safety.

The treatment plan   should be based on each individual's goals and needs to address the   deficits that diminish that person's ability to communicate efficiently and effectively. It should build   upon and exploit strengths.   Treatment implementation should   be accompanied by data collection to assess the effectiveness of the treatments.

Another important element in the treatment of adults with RHD is counseling family members and caregivers about   a patient's abilities and deficits, especially since these cognitive-communicative deficits are often   unfamiliar to the general population. Speech-language pathologists also   serve as case managers to coordinate   and ensure appropriate and timely delivery of a management plan

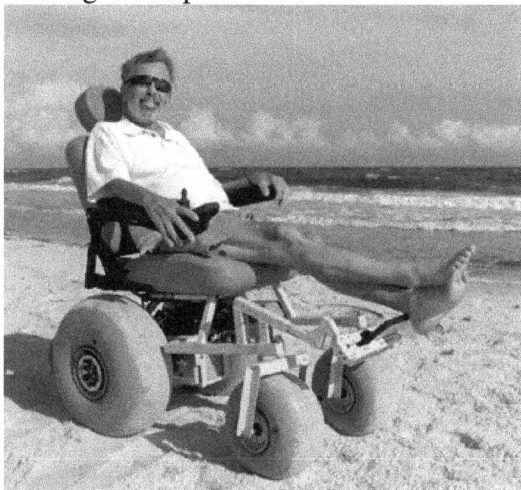

↳Life can be fun if you have appropriate equipment.

.

What is Wrong With Hospice

In general, patients must meet the following criteria to be eligible for hospice care:

- Adults with a prognosis of six months or less if the disease runs its normal course
- A prognosis that is certified by the patient's primary care physician as well as the hospice medical director
- Both the patient and family desire palliative care as opposed to curative treatment *[Author's 12-year companion, Steven Lee Hatch, the patient, was not asked if he was ready for hospice. That is where laws were broken. As long as he could answer "yes" or "no" to simple questions, his answer was required before taking him out of skilled curative treatment and placed into palliative care (sedatives/morphine). He died just 13 days after being forced into hospice. MJW]*
- Hospice can continue beyond six months as long as the patient continues to meet eligibility criteria

Is it too early?

A common misconception about hospice care is that a referral can be premature. Hospice care is most effective over a period of months, yet most hospice patients die within a month of referral based on the reluctance to refer patients earlier.

An early referral can provide your residents with the extra attention and focused hospice care that relieves symptoms and manages pain. It also offers your individuals and their families a vital opportunity to deal with their loss and say goodbye.

[NOTE: Author disagrees with referral to earlier-than-needed hospice care after a <u>stroke</u>. Strokes have a long recovery period. Once in hospice, the stroke victim will no longer receive therapy or rehabilitation. If you want to <u>get rid of your unloved one</u> who had a stroke, put them in hospice right away and they will soon die in their sleep!

The majority of stroke victims live and most want to live even if they will have some sign of their disability for the rest of their lives. Just remember, you might be the next stroke victim who will be allowed to die early just because you have a disability from a stroke.

To enter hospice is your decision, no one can legally place you in hospice without your permission. If you can answer "yes" or "no" or even blink your eyelid, your permission can not be overridden. You have a right to live and to have therapy/rehabilitation to recover. MJW]

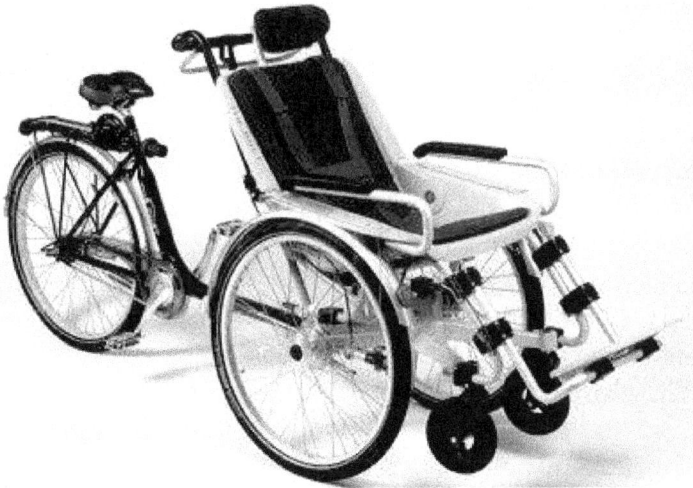

Bicycle to take your loved one for a ride.

Illnesses Causing 100% Inability to Communicate

The term "locked-in syndrome" was first introduced in 1966 to describe a state in which a patient is locked inside their body, able to perceive their situation, but with extremely limited ability for interaction. Patients recount that the worst aspect of this syndrome is the anxious desire to move or speak while being unable to do so.

Locked-in syndrome (LIS), also known as cerebromedullospinal disconnection, de-efferented state or pseudocoma, is a rare neurological disorder in which there is complete paralysis of all voluntary movements except movements of the eyes – vertical gaze and eyelid opening.

In classical LIS, unlike coma or the vegetative state, individuals are conscious, alert and awake; there is often no impairment of language, memory and intellectual functions; sensation is sometimes also preserved. Due to the loss of voluntary movements, speech is also lost. Communication may be possible through eye movements or blinking.

Incomplete LIS can occur when there are remnants of voluntary movements; total LIS, on the other hand, consists of complete immobility, including loss of eye movements, while maintaining consciousness.

The most common cause for LIS is a lesion in the pons, a part of the brainstem that contains nerve fibers that relay information to other areas of the brain, usually due to brainstem stroke. Another relatively frequent cause is traumatic brain injury, either directly by brainstem lesions or secondary to vascular damage or occlusion. Other, less frequent causes have been reported such as brainstem tumor or brainstem drug toxicity, for example. Another important cause of complete LIS can be observed in end-stage amyotrophic lateral sclerosis (ALS), a motor neuron disease.

The first person to realize the patient is conscious is often a family member. LIS diagnosis can sometimes take months or even years, since signs of consciousness may not always be easily or immediately perceptible. For a long time, LIS was actually mostly diagnosed retrospectively based on postmortem findings. Unless the physician is aware of the signs and symptoms of LIS, the patient may incorrectly be considered to be in a coma or vegetative state.

Electroencephalographic (EEG) recordings in patients with LIS are usually normal or minimally altered and show reactivity to external stimuli. The presence of a relatively normal reactive EEG rhythm in a patient that appears to be unconscious can allow the diagnosis of LIS. Functional neuroimaging tools, namely PET imaging and functional MRI (fMRI) have shown sensitivity for identification of patients in a minimally conscious state, and may become useful tools to complement bedside examinations.

Individuals with LIS can survive for significant periods of time. Although most deaths occur in the first four months. Once a patient has medically stabilized for more than a year, 10 year survival is 83% and 20 year survival is 40%. However, there is no cure or standard treatment available. Typically, the motor rehabilitation is very limited, although some control of fingers and toe movements may be recovered, often allowing a functional use of a digital switch.

Communication can be achieved by a code using eyelid blinks or vertical eye movements. The simplest form can be a yes/no code, such as looking up, indicating "yes" and looking down indicating "no." A higher level of communication may be achieved through alphabetical systems that allow patients to indicate a letter through eye movement, thereby building sentences. This has even allowed books to be written by LIS patients.

Jean-Dominique Bauby, editor-in-chief of the fashion magazine Elle, had a brainstem stroke in December 1995, at the age of 43. After several weeks in a coma, he emerged into LIS, only able to move his left eyelid. Bauby, wanting to share his experience with the world, dictated a book that he composed mentally. Each passage was dictated letter by letter using a frequency-ordered alphabet with Bauby choosing letters by blinking. His book *The Diving Bell and the Butterfly* was published two days before his death in March 1997 and became a best-seller. The book was later adapted into a film of the same name, released in 2007.

Other firsthand accounts of living with LIS include *Look Up for Yes* (1997), by Julia Tavalaro, and *Only the Eyes Say Yes* (1997), by Philippe Vigand.

Julia Tavalaro fell into a coma after a hemorrhage in 1966, at the age of 32. After seven months, she woke up in a chronic care facility where she was regarded as a "vegetable". It was only after several years that her family noticed a smile as a reaction to a dirty joke. She initially communicated using a letter board, but later used a communication device to write poetry, and managed to cheek-control her wheelchair. She died in 2003 at the age of 68.

Philippe Vigand fell into a coma in 1990 due to a vertebral artery dissection, also at the age of 32. He remained in a coma for two months and was later treated as a "vegetable". His wife eventually noticed him blinking in response to her questions, but was unable to convince the treating physicians of his conscious state. His speech therapist was able to diagnose LIS when Vigand grinned after an insult from the therapist, whose finger was bitten by Vigand while testing his gag reflex. He then asked how much two plus two was and Vigand blinked four times confirming his cognitive capacities. He initially also communicated using a letter board, but later used an infrared camera attached to a computer.

Meanwhile, technology has contributed significantly to patients' communication abilities. Instruments such as infra-red eye movement sensors coupled to virtual keyboards allow the use of word processors which in turn can be coupled to a text-to-speech synthesizer. These can also let the LIS patient control his environment, access the Internet and use e-mail, for example. Brain-computer interfaces (BCI) are also tools that allow LIS patients to control devices directly, but by using

EEG signals to control computers. An example is the use of BCI involving visual presentation of letters associated with selection through EEG and a statistical language model. However, these tools are mostly still being tested or are too expensive for generalized use.

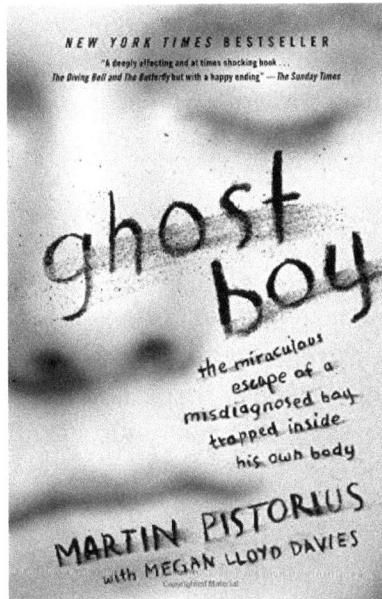

NEW YORK TIMES BESTSELLER
"A deeply affecting and at times shocking book . . .
The Diving Bell and The Butterfly but with a happy ending" — The Sunday Times

ghost boy
the miraculous escape of a misdiagnosed boy trapped inside his own body

MARTIN PISTORIUS
with MEGAN LLOYD DAVIES

An easy to read true story. *Ghost Boy,* was written by Martin Pistorius who was a normal child. He suffered an illness that spread to his brain and caused him to become a mute quadriplegic. By his fourteenth birthday he was a hollow shell, unseeing and unknowing, he spent his days at a care center, sitting blankly in front of the TV while his family waited for him to die.

Then his mind began to return but for ten torturous years he was unable to get anyone to realize the boy had returned since his body was still non-reactive to his commands. While the boy/man in this story is more severe than a stroke victim who usually can make eye contact, smile on one side of their mouth, can utter sounds similar to "yes" and "no" plus move one side of their body, this man only regained a limited ability to move his body or to speak. He not only returned to an active life as functioning person but became employed and even married.

[Author's note: I added the above examples of people who had no ability to communicate for years yet eventually were able to communicate. It is much easier to determine if a stroke victim's mind is normal. Steve Hatch was able to answer "yes" and "no" appropriately to caregiver's questions plus he made eye-contact and could respond with his non-paralyzed left hand including shaking hands.

Yet a doctor who had never seen Steve before July 24th, ran no tests on him, called him a "vegetable" after he was revived from fainting after a 30-minute van ride, then recommended he be placed in Hospice without asking him. Iowa law clearly states that a conscious person cannot be placed into hospice without their permission. That was Steven Lee Hatch's death sentence. MJW]

This following statement was found on the internet with a 3-minute search. I saved the link and only offer one paragraph from the news article. I'm not the only one who has uncovered a "death for profit" scam though this one did not happen in Iowa.

"Hospice is a for-profit business that is under investigation in multiple states for breaking laws. The U.S. Department of Justice sued several hospices for milking, or bilking, Medicare for millions of dollars—in some cases by **enrolling elderly patients who were not terminally ill.** A blistering investigation uncovered sales contests and high-pressure marketing tactics at a few for-profits—including a "Christmas Cash Blitz," a "Fall Frenzy," and a "September Sizzle" at a hospice that paid employees as much as $100 a head for referrals."

Stroke Survivor's Prayer

God, I come before You as one whose injury
cannot be seen by your other children.

While others see me, they know not that
my wounds are invisible.

I come before you as a
Traumatic brain injury survivor.

You alone know the depth of my pain,
of my despair, my confusion, my aloneness,
And my overwhelming loss of self.

When others leave my life, help me to
remember that You are always there with me.

When unsteadiness causes me to stumble,
please take my hand and lead me safely forward.

While my memory so often fails me,
help me to never forget what is really important.

God, so many of your children walk daily with
challenges that dwarf my own.

By understanding this, I can see my own
life in a better perspective.

Help me for today to accept my fate in this life
knowing that if I trust in you, all will be well.
Amen.

His Spirit Fights Back

The Premature Death of
Steven Lee Hatch
July 13, 1948 - August 6, 2015

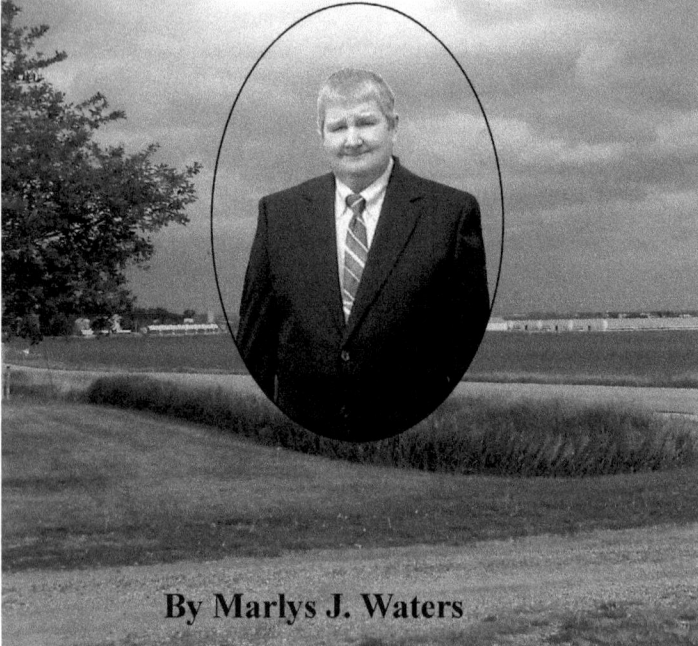

By Marlys J. Waters

About the Author

Marlys J. (Launspach) Waters was born and raised on a farm southeast of Nemaha, Iowa. After graduating from Crestland Community School (Early and Nemaha) in 1963, she attended Iowa State University and Drake University, and stayed thirty years in the Ames and Des Moines area.

Marlys returned to her hometown of Nemaha, Iowa in 1993 to care for her parents. She now manages two online bookstores, runs a used book and music store, hosts local websites, and writes books.

Steven Lee Hatch, was three years younger than Marlys and their family farms were only four miles apart. The pair finally connected 40 years later -- a friendship that spanned twelve years and was comprised of hobby farming together with a variety of livestock, assorted antique farm machinery and tractors plus harvesting Steve's large garden.

Steve's death shortly after his stroke was the motivation for the publication of this book that speaks for the person who was silenced and to promote a better understanding of strokes and recovery. Post-stroke life can return to normal with a willing invalid and his companion to make it happen. But Steve wasn't allowed to choose his care nor his caregiver.

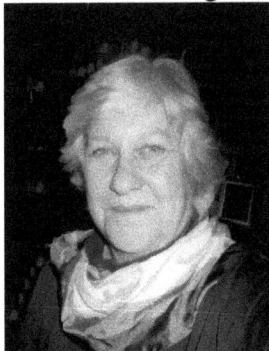

CPSIA information can be obtained
at www.ICGtesting.com
Printed in the USA
BVHW01s1749110218
507833BV00012B/229/P

9 781530 787586